MOM

Mehra's Orthopedics for MCI

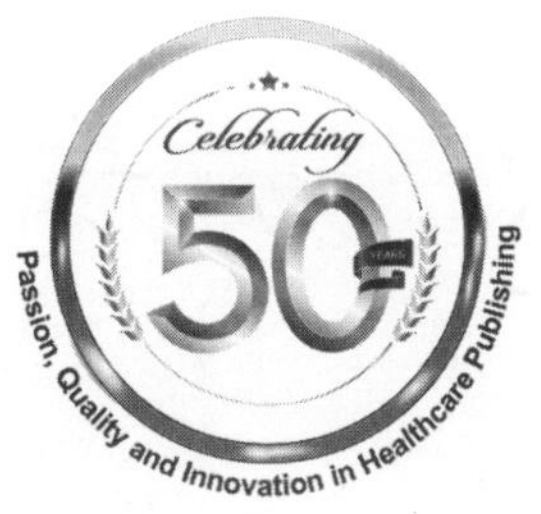

MOM

Mehra's Orthopedics for MCI

Second Edition

Apurv Mehra
MBBS MAMC MS ORTHO (UCMS)
DNB ORTHO DIP. SICOT, (Belgium)
Fellowship Computer Navigation Joint Replacement
from Germany, Australia and Malaysia

Consultant Orthopedic Surgeon
Computer Navigation Joint Replacement
and Arthroscopy Surgeon

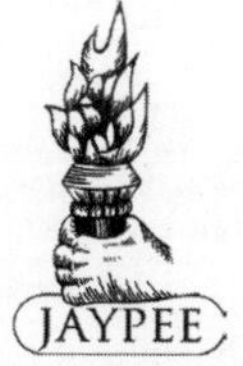

JAYPEE BROTHERS MEDICAL PUBLISHERS

The Health Sciences Publisher

New Delhi | London | Panama

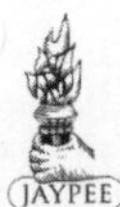

Jaypee Brothers Medical Publishers (P) Ltd.

Headquarters
Jaypee Brothers Medical Publishers (P) Ltd
4838/24, Ansari Road, Daryaganj
New Delhi 110 002, India
Phone: +91-11-43574357
Fax: +91-11-43574314
E-mail: jaypee@jaypeebrothers.com

Overseas Offices
J.P. Medical Ltd
83, Victoria Street, London
SW1H 0HW (UK)
Phone: +44 20 3170 8910
Fax: +44 (0)20 3008 6180
E-mail: info@jpmedpub.com

Jaypee-Highlights Medical Publishers Inc
City of Knowledge, Bld. 235, 2nd Floor, Clayton
Panama City, Panama
Phone: +1 507-301-0496
Fax: +1 507-301-0499
E-mail: cservice@jphmedical.com

Jaypee Brothers Medical Publishers (P) Ltd
Bhotahity, Kathmandu, Nepal
Phone: +977-9741283608
E-mail: kathmandu@jaypeebrothers.com

Website: www.jaypeebrothers.com
Website: www.jaypeedigital.com

Inquiries for bulk sales may be solicited at: jaypee@jaypeebrothers.com

MOM - Mehra's Orthopedics for MCI

First Edition: 2015

Second Edition: **2018**

ISBN: 978-93-5270-584-9

Printed at Rajkamal Electric Press, Kundli, Haryana.

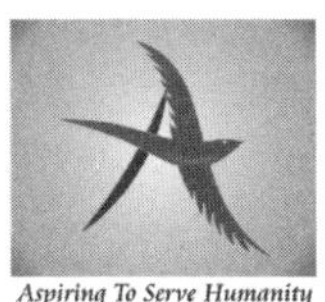

Mission

Aspiring to Serve Humanity

Invest In Your Dreams!
Grind Now... Shine Later!!!

This book is dedicated to

My Daughter, Vrinda Mehra
My Patients & My Students who have helped me evolve as an Orthopedic Surgeon & a Teacher

— Dr. Apurv Mehra

"People are often unreasonable and self-centered. Forgive them anyway. If you are kind, people may accuse you of ulterior motives. Be kind anyway. If you are honest, people may cheat you. Be honest anyway. If you find happiness, people may be jealous. Be happy anyway. The good you do today may be forgotten tomorrow. Do good anyway. Give the world the best you have and it may never be enough. Give your best anyway. For you see, in the end, it is between you and God.

— Mother Teresa

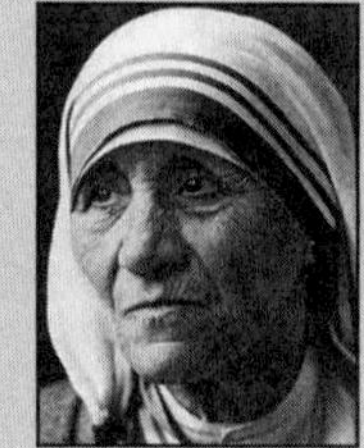

Preface

I extend my heartfelt gratitude to all my students for the wonderful response given to the previous edition of MOM.

MOM became a favorite of all FMGE Students in the very first edition. The credit of MOM's instant recognition owes to Ortho Pedics Quick Review (OPQR) for being 'The Best Seller' MCQ Book for Orthopedics for PG preparation. The success of Ortho Pedics Quick Review created an instant demand to come up with a mini version of OPQR exclusively for FMGE Students.

MOM Second edition is a small book that explains the basics of Orthopedics in a very simple manner, precisely for FMG Students.

Unique Selling Points:

The biggest strength of this book is its simplicity - All Concepts explained in simple manner

- More concise, more compact and more comprehensive for easy understanding.
- More illustrated diagrams and lots of new images for better retention
- Includes new flowcharts and new mnemonics for easier recall during examinations
- New topics added as per the latest MCI guidelines and trends in exams
- Special Chapter 'Summary of Orthopedics' to revise complete orthopedics in just few hours before exam.

— Dr. Apurv Mehra

Mail Your Queries @Orthopedicsquickreview@gmail.com
Lets Connect @ Facebook: Apurv Mehra
Get Inspired : www.drapurv.com

GOOD THINGS TAKE TIME...

Here are Answers to Few Questions I Am Often Asked by My Students...

Q. 1. Why didn't I achieve a rank when I worked so hard...?

My Answer: I would like to share with you, when most of my friends qualified in the first attempt and I didn't, it was a heartbreak and quite unbelievable. That is when I realized that our so called failure in entrance exams is not a failure but is the inability to plan a strategy and identify our areas of lacunae.

I analyzed my lacunas & came to this conclusion:

- Group all 19 subjects into 4 parts
  - Part 1:-First year subjects
  - Part 2:-Second Year Subjects
  - Part 3:- Final year subjects including PSM
  - Part 4:-Short subjects that include skin, Psychiatry, Radio, Anaesthesia, ENT, Optha, Ortho & Forensic Medicine
- After assessing last 5 year papers, on the basis of my MCQ knowledge I noted
  - My weak subjects, Strong Subjects & Relatively Strong Subjects
  - In my weak subjects, I made a list of topics to be covered and
  - In my relatively better subjects, I made a list of topics I was weak in.

This is a point that we need to understand & accept that even in our strong subjects there will be areas we are weak in.

A good player of cricket is the one who needs to be a good runner but if his running is weak then he'll be run out, so he needs to work on his running. As well at the same time he needs to keep practicing his batting skills too.

Through this I wish to convey that you should keep revising your strengths otherwise soon they become your short comings .

Q. 2. Why do we keep forgetting what we learn...?

My Answer: In your first reading itself, make it a habit to highlight important points to be read in your second reading. This helps you a lot In the second reading as it gives you a feel that you have already read this earlier & also saves your time.

I also advice to make 2 schedules:

1. Main schedule for preparation for the whole day.
2. Revision Schedule in which you have 90 minutes each day to revise volatile subjects, for example for me - Pharma was one such subject.

Q. 3. Why do we lag behind in our schedule ...?

My Answer: You can never complete 100% of any subject. Selective Study is the best way to prepare for Medical Entrance Exams.

Read each subject in the order of importance of the topics so that in case you exceed your time allotted to each subject, you move on to the next subject but don't miss on vital things. Here our aim is to complete all 19 subjects. But if you till the end don't follow this advice of sticking with your schedule, you will end up with a catastrophe of leaving a subject which no one can never compensate.

Also keep practicing MCQ's every day, preferably in the morning hours, at the same time when the exams are conducted, so that your internal clock is tuned .

Q. 4. Negative Thoughts- What if I study properly and still don't make it this time then what ...???

My Answer: There is a self-belief which tells you to take chances. I agree there will be doubts but you must at the same time realize that even Rank 1 of any exam, will have doubts but even then the power to conquer the fears is more. So the basic thing you can do to counter this is - to develop a habit of surrounding yourself with positivity and positive human beings and to my brain, they are your parents- talk to them, they will always show you the positive aspect .

Q. 5. Sir, when will my time come...?

My Answer: This is a big question and I can just tell you one simple thing. 'Time never comes, you need to create it.' God will write your destiny according to your efforts, and only hard work can beat any talent and I know it surely will.

My batchmates in MAMC were very talented and intelligent but I always had this habit called as hard work, which I gradually realized is the biggest asset, which if nurtured and fed well, can take you everywhere. Those who work hard can do good not only with themselves but also to lots of people around. Just as I have learnt from my Grandmother, 'To live like a king, we need to work like a slave.'

So to summarise:

- Right approach to examination is the most important step, so start as early as you can.
- Select the right books with updated pretexts in latest editions.
- Your preparation decides your fate, analyze and evaluate your current preparation.
- Accordingly start with a combo of strong & weak subjects. Prepare list of important topics, shortlist topics in weak subjects and weak topics in strong subjects.
- Be consistent and keep revising your strong topics too at the same time managing your time well.
- Practice MCQ's daily, preferably from the topics you have read.
- Plan your day in advance to bring in effectiveness.
- Prepare a schedule where you also give 90 minutes to revision each day.
- Stick to your time table and don't neglect any subject- completing all subjects is more important than trying to complete 100 per cent of a subject.
- Keep talking to your parents, they are the sea of positivity and will always stand by you.
- Hard work can beat talent, it surely will, so work hard like a slave and then live like a king.

FOR MY PATRIOTS

A Message from My Heart...

First of all, pat your back and be proud to be a 'Doctor' the most noble profession on earth. You are an achiever and are now preparing for a bigger challenge...Indian PG Medical Entrance Exam which is bound to become more difficult with each passing year with the rise in the number of individuals appearing for these entrance exams every year.

I, Dr. Apurv Mehra, Your Teacher, take it as my responsibility to guide and help you achieve what you desire.

First & Foremost:

To turn your dreams into reality, there is NO SHORT CUT, instead all you need to do is:

- Draw a plan for the next day before you sleep so that by the time you get up, you already have a target to achieve.
- Study **SIX hours** per day without your mobile phone, for a period of six months.
- Always remember, selections in Entrance Exams are not based on intelligence or knowledge, but on more number of revisions of important topics & following a proper strategy
- Prepare notes, crisp & easy for you to understand, only if you are going to use them for revision. Otherwise it's just a waste of time.!!
- Go for selective reading of important topics (follow General Rule), practice MCQ'S, do refer to standard text books for concepts/doubts/controversies.
- Prepare your own small diary of mnemonics, powerful enough for you to remember.

A combined approach is a must to prepare for all Entrance Exams (NEET DNB /AIIMS/ PGI / JIPMER)

- It is advisable to go through last 7 years AIIMS papers, 6-8 PGI papers & 3 - 4 DNB papers.
- Memorize the important topics of last 5 years All India questions. Don't forget to check recent updates.

- Revise your notes you have made and also course notes if you had joined any coaching institute.
- No need to waste time on finding answers to controversial questions just decide an answer you will mark if asked in exam.
- Your knowledge & presence of mind are equally important on the day of the exam.
- Make use of every single day. (Read, Practice, Revise)
- Keep a positive attitude throughout.

Do not count the days make the days count!

10 lessons I learnt in my journey of starting from nowhere...just nowhere...

1. Attitude...

Life may not have given you enough reasons but smile and also laugh and do both every often. After this just pause and think the difference between smile and laugh....

2. Struggle...

The fight for the victory is more precious than the victory and most important is the attitude in handling the fight and the victory....

3. Supporters...

The supporters are like noose around your neck that can only constrict you or stop you just untie and release them as soon as possible....and then jump and fly...

4. Success...

First success is just the declaration of your arrival and then progress on your journey...

5. Failure...

Everyone knows how to handle success, precious is to handle failure with the same grace and then just announce you failed ...but have the courage to turn it into success...have the courage to standup for yourself...

6. Planning...

Plan and also most importantly execute the plan...

7. Innovative...

Be innovative and be conceptual....and have the courage to follow your conceptual innovation...

8. Thoughts about business...

Refusal in any business is to reject a possible growth plan and acceptance in business is about the expenditure whereas success is about the precarious balance between the refusal and acceptance....

9. My career...

Most felt I was not good enough to do MS Orthopedics, Most felt I could not teach as they claimed that I was not gifted with that talent.... but they did not measure my hard work and determination and with those I could defeat the talent. Most importantly they did not realize it was my dream and I wanted to live that dream badly and there was good God above ... rest was history...

10. Always remember these two most important things - Thirst and Hunger are for your soul, so take care that it is fed well...

FEW VALUABLE PEARLS THAT SHALL HELP YOU ALWAYS

A Day Before The Examination

Every time we would go to write an exam our seniors (at MAMC) would tell to us....

1. Sleep on time and sleep well a night before.
2. Before sleeping preferably speak to your closest family member or your wise friend and do promise that you will give your best and keep a positive attitude.
3. Reading few jokes from a joke book has been found as a stress reliever by some.
4. On the morning of the exam, never go empty stomach never eat too much, take a balanced fruit, a sandwich and a cup of coffee/tea is preferred by most.
5. Always get ready on time and wear your most comfortable clothes and shoes. Trying out a new footwear is not advisable.
6. Most prefer some music in morning hours to de-stress themselves.
7. Leave early from house for the center and avoid driving at any cost.
8. Make sure to carry your Photo Identity proof, Admit card and Stationary.
9. At the center preferably involve yourself in some meditation or stay with your family or friend accompanying you. Avoid mingling with groups.
10. Please do all the formalities before the exam on time to avoid any last minute panic.
11. Follow instructions of the examiners or invigilators at the center dare not involve in any of them

On The Day Of The Exam

TELL YOURSELF... IF I CAN'T NO ONE CAN...

Remember to take up challenges...

Each day the heart has fear, each day the mind has doubts, for most of us it's a big issue... but for few it's a challenge...

- Outside the examination hall there are three different kinds of student personalities.
  - Category 1) Geared and charged up, discussing things in over excited manner. You will find them discussing all the important things and their BMR too is toned up –that's the **Hyper Group**.

- Category 2) **The Quiet Group** revising and reading in a corner. On their faces you will find serenity and shine, they are not talking or mingling with anyone, they are just with their notes.
- Category 3) **The Analyst Group** is calm & quite. They have no book in their hand & are just sitting in a corner planning their exam strategy, reminding themselves that they have actually worked hard for this exam and now they need to carefully select out the questions.

- Category of questions asked in every entrance exam:-
  - The first category of questions are the ones you already know about (Repeat Questions) and You should try to get all of them correct- Please read carefully & go slow on them.
  - The second category of questions will be the ones which will require you to make educated guesses, questions which you already will have some idea about. Such questions require time –PAY ATTENTION & CAREFULLY ANSWER THEM
  - The third category of questions will be the new ones which most of the students will find tough to answer but if you try to find out the answer by carefully ruling out the options it might help.

The Analyst is the group that understands their preparation can never be completed 100 per cent so studying outside the examination hall will not make much of a difference (Just Like category 1 or category 2 students).

- Outside the hall is the place to fill yourself with positivity & encouragement alongwith a well-planned strategy.(Category 3)
- Remember strategy is always more powerful than knowledge and talent.
- Stay calm, even those who Top don't know everything, but they apply all the knowledge that they know, they plan their strategies and they plan well.

Finally your results will depend on the strategies you followed ...
So enter the examination hall with positivity , well planned strategy and self belief...**If I can't no one else can... Believe in yourself...it really works...**

During The Exam...

- Start the paper and read each question very carefully.
- Oneliners should be read at least 3 times and message should be very clear what the examiner is asking and then read all 4 choices.
- One by one try to rule out options so that you have more probability of getting the answers correct for e.g: If you select one answer out of 4 then your success probability is 25% but if you rule out one option then your success probability is 33% and if you are able to rule out 2 options then you have to mark from the remaining 2 choices thus your success probability is 50%.
- Do not make a mistake of marking the first answer without reading all 4 choices. Most of the examiners set 3 to 4 % questions on the principle that student marks the first answer on reflex.

This makes a total of about 10 to 12 questions in your exam thus can make a huge difference.

- Please do not try to find mistakes in questions. For all practical reasons try to answer questions accepting them as correctly framed.
- Multiple lines or clinical questions should be answered on remembering the following points:
  - Age of the patient may help you decide the answer.
  - Unilateral or bilateral may help you rule out few choices
  - Normal features mentioned helps rule out few choices
  - Please make a note of important radiological findings.
  - Give very high importance to histopathological or biopsy features to arrive at diagnosis and always give tissue diagnosis more importance than radiological findings because radiological finding can be non-specific.
  - Always make a note whether most common finding is asked or most characteristic finding is asked.
  - Similarly observe that whether investigation of choice is asked or gold standard investigation is asked.
  - If you look at questions, investigation of choice refers to next investigation and gold standard refers to best investigation usually.
- Each question is highly valuable and do not take any question lightly no matter how much confident you are.
- It is very strange that students try to save time on the questions that they have knowledge about and give more time to questions they are not aware of. Actually you must focus strongly on topics you know and answer their questions carefully rather than giving more time to topics you are unaware of. Most Toppers get the repeat topics correct as compared to scoring high on new topics.

My Grand Mother used to recite these Lines from Guru Granth Sahib...... which I often read out to all My students.

"Teri kismat da likha
Teretoh koi khonahinsakda
Tushram (Karam) karachalbande...
Je usdimeher hove ta tenu o v mil jaugajotera ho nahinsakda"

Go Chase Your Dreams, I Pray To Almighty To Grant It...!!!

—Dr. Apurv Mehra

your queries – orthodhoomdhadaka@gmail.com
Let's Connect @ Apurv Mehra (Profile 1, 2 or 3) OR Apurv Mehra
Get Inspired @ www.drapurv.com

ORTHO DHOOM DHADAKA (ODD)

India's Leading Orthopedics Lecture By Dr. Apurv Mehra

(For UG & PG Aspirants Preparing for AIIMS/AIPG NEET/PGI/DNB & JIPMER)

Ortho Dhoom Dhadaka (ODD), India's leading Lecture on Orthopedics is a highly successful program conducted by Dr. Apurv Mehra. Ortho Dhoom Dhadaka (ODD) is not just about Orthopedics but goes beyond that, as Dr. Apurv Mehra believes that education should be fun as well as inspiring.

Born on 14th August, 2014, ODD is a dream come true and is a landmark in history. Standing true to its name, Ortho Dhoom Dhadaka (Dhoom Dhadaka means a gala event) within three months achieved grand success, not only by going house full in all the cities it was organized, but more importantly by the recognition, its name has received, is one of its kind in the world of Medical Education.

Ortho Dhoom Dhadaka is a humble initiative by Dr. Apurv Mehra to strengthen his bond with his students & help them achieve their goals. Inspired from his lectures, students not only 'learn' but actually follow Dr. Apurv Mehra and also implement his advice & guidance in their day to day lives.

Dr. Apurv Mehra provides the vision and high content resources needed to take students to the next level. Hundreds of students have benefitted from his dynamic lectures.

DR APURV MEHRA–THE ORTHOPEDIC SURGEON

Dr. Apurv Mehra is an Internationally Trained & Experienced Computer Navigation Joint Replacement & Arthroscopy Surgeon. He is an Orthopedic Consultant at Max Institute of Bone & Joint Care at Patparganj, Delhi. Dr. Apurv Mehra is the Founder & Director of Vidya Jeevan Ortho Pedics Centre, Delhi -India's most Trusted Orthopedic Centre as per Leading Clinicians.

He has exceptional academic skills, his clear logical thoughts and approach to Complex surgical issues makes him a standout in Knee

Arthoplasty and Ligament Reconstructions. Thereby helping his patients to return back to sports activities. His clinical skills are exemplary, he achieves good outcomes, and his patients love him.

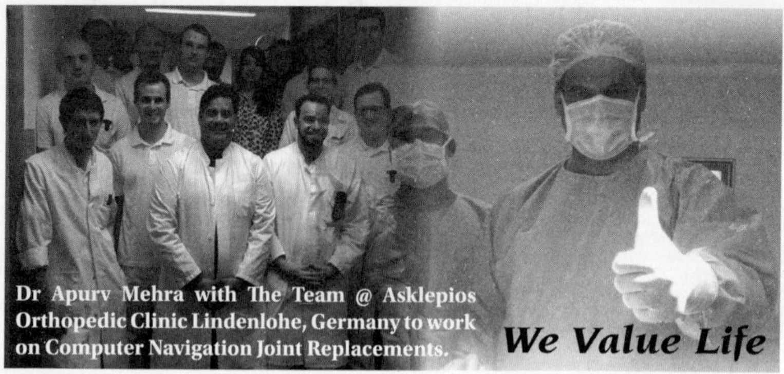

Dr Apurv Mehra with The Team @ Asklepios Orthopedic Clinic Lindenlohe, Germany to work on Computer Navigation Joint Replacements.

MEDMIRACLE: EMPOWERS TO EXCEL

MedMiracle - Online Guide To Help You In PG Preparation

MedMiracle is an initiative to provide students preparing for PG Entrance Exams - handy tricks & tips, logical approach on 'How to study' 19 subjects, useful revision strategies based on concrete concepts & 'Must know' things through videos & other methods that will add an extra edge to their PG Preparation.

MedMiracle is a Team of Leading Educationists, Group of Passionate Students (PG Toppers from The Best Institutes & 19 Subject Specialists. Our solo aim here @ MedMiracle is to make this arduous journey of PG Entrance easier, with specific and comprehensive content to bridge the gap between what we read & what is being tested so as to help each student crack these ever-changing PG Entrance Examinations with ease.

What is MedMiracle

MedMiracle is the shortest and strongest bridge between demand & supply of a technology that can help medical students perform better during their postgraduate entrance exams and MBBS professionals.

MedMiracle understands that PG Aspirants require a helping hand to master the vast pool of 19 subjects. Hence it is creating a conglomerate of content to provide directional studies to retain the affection to the beauty called 'Medicine.'

Medmiracle aims to gradually become the shadow of every medico and at the same time make sure that it provides help to propel their career against the winds of competition.

MedMiracle is the one stop answer to everything you need to know, when it matters the most.

We are not here to only draw guidelines. We are a flexible group who will plan custom made roadways helping in reaching destinations, depending upon strength & weakness of every PG aspirant.

Working Principle of MedMiracle

MedMiracle follows The 80:20 Rule : How to spend less time studying yet be more productive. We all know how it feels to be inefficient: spending many hours studying without getting much productive work done can be incredibly frustrating, and is a drain on time and energy for students everywhere.

What if you could spend LESS time studying, but still get MORE done in your day? If this sounds too good to be true, then prepare to be pleasantly surprised. With the help of MedMiracle -Tests, Note & Audio -Video Lessons 80% of your exam success will come from 20% of the work you put in.

Story Behind MedMiracle

Being in the Medical Teaching Industry for more than two decades, we have witnessed tremendous changes in the PG Medical Entrance Exams. We realized there was only ONE GOAL that each budding yet struggling doctor was aiming for and that was A PG SEAT. In order to get this PG Seat, all they needed was PROPER GUIDANCE and LOGICAL SOLUTIONS to help them achieve the same, not merely for the reason to earn a living but also to justify their decision of getting into the most noble profession on earth.

To come across as a genuine help, We- A Team of Leading Educationists, Subject specialists and group of Passionate Students (PG Toppers from the best institutes) have joined together to form MEDMIRACLE–An Online Support Group to guide students preparing for the Postgraduate Examinations like NEET, AIIMS, PGI and JIPMER.

MedMiracle App—Empowers To Excel

To help Every PG Aspirant realize their dream in the most easiest way, MedMiracle has developed offerings catering to students needs:

- Test Series with Detailed Performance Analysis
- MCQ Bank -Evaluation System Based On Real PG Entrance Exams
- Exam Oriented Personalised Notes
- Audio & Video Lessons on difficult topics of all 19 subjects
- Time Based Customised Schedules
- Daily Revisions through Multimodal Teachings - Important Pearls

Medicine is a branch of wonders. We @ MedMiracle shall reignite students' zeal and make learning a great new experience!!!

Contents

Chapter 1

Imaging for Orthopedics

Orthopaedics: The term was coined by **Nicolas Andry**. Orthos means straight and paedics means child so orthopaedics means **Straight child.**

Definition of orthopaedics: The branch of surgery that deals with the prevention or correction of injuries or disorders of the skeletal system and associated muscles, joints and ligaments.

ROLE OF IMAGING IN ORTHOPAEDICS

A. X-rays are usually the first radiological investigation done in orthopaedics and its uses involves Screening of Cortex and Marrow. **X-rays are the first investigations in traumatic disorders**.

- Glass pieces are visualized on X-rays.

Soft tissue planes (muscle and fat planes) are visualised on X-rays and often students forget this!

(Loss of soft tissue planes is earliest X-ray changes in infection/swelling in limb and it is seen after 24–48 hours of onset of disease, they are more useful for infections than tumors).

Cartilage is not seen on X-rays

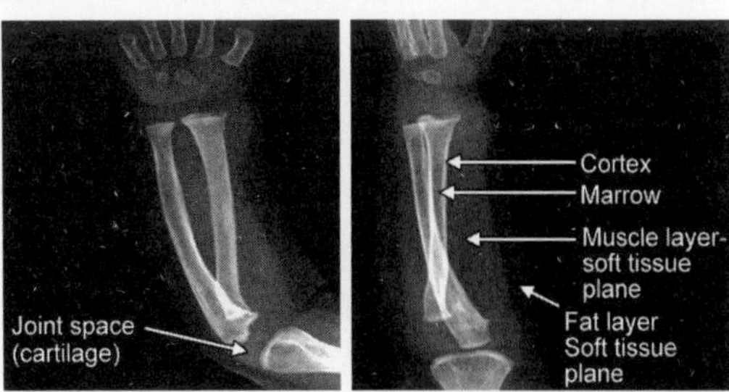

Fig. 1.1: X-ray of forearm with wrist with elbow

Note: Joint space is a misnomer, Actually there is no space in areas of joints, **it is the cartilage occupied area** which is not visualised on X-ray. Thus whenever joint is destroyed, cartilage is destroyed hence joint space is reduced on X-rays.

Types of Periosteal Reaction : Periosteal Reaction : Indicates Bone Damage

1. *No reaction:* **Tuberculosis of bones does not usually have a periosteal reaction.**
2. Narrow zone of activity e.g. Solid periosteal reaction (single layer of periosteal elevation) is seen in benign lesion like.
   a. **Benign tumors or Pyogenic Osteomyelitis**
   b. In case of osteomyelitis the periosteal reaction is seen on day 7 to 10th (or 2nd week or day 10th)

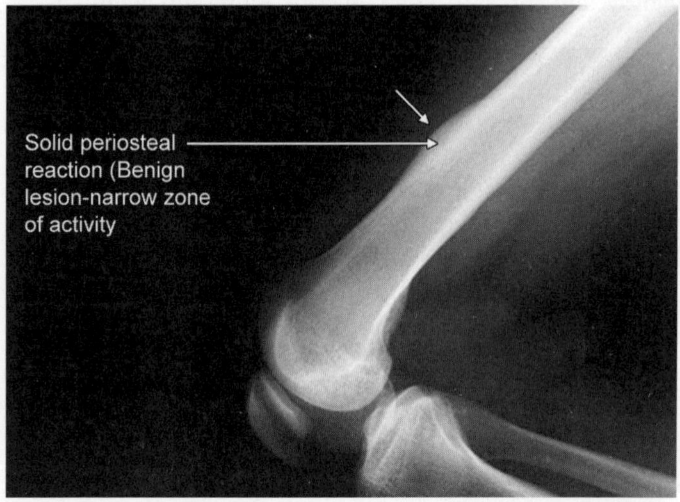

Fig. 1.2: Solid periosteal reaction

3. In **malignant lesions** there is wide area of activity e.g. Onion peel/codmans triangle and sunray appearance (all are indicative of wide area of activity).
   a. Onion peel or lamellated appearance—Seen in any malignant or chronic lesions (e.g. chronic osteomyelitis) but usually ewings sarcoma.

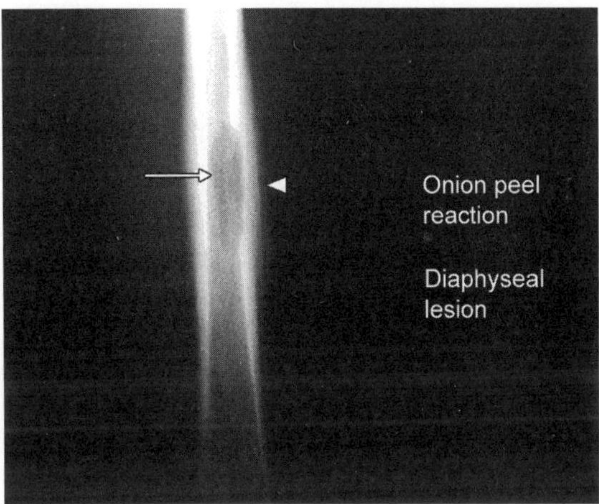

Fig. 1.3: Onion peel reaction

b. **Codman Triangle:** Triangular bone growth seen at angle of lifting of periosteum; it can be seen in any malignant lesion but usually osteosarcoma.

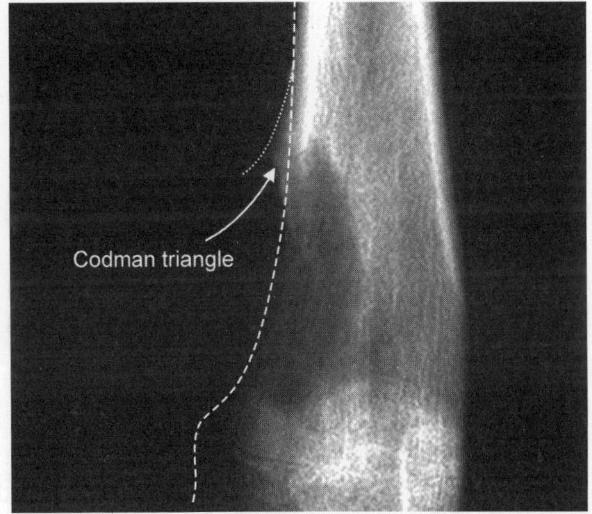

Fig. 1.4: Codman triangle

c. **Sunray appearance**/sunburst/spiculated appearance – can be seen in **any malignant lesion** but usually **osteosarcoma**.

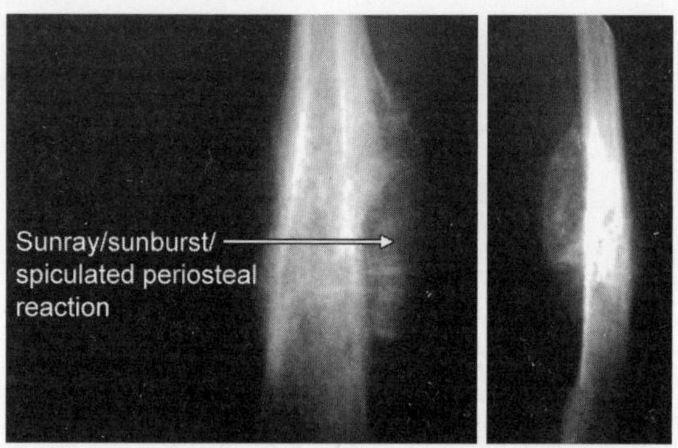

Fig. 1.5: Sunray appearance

B. **CT Scan:** CT Scan is the investigation for cortex and calcification.

C. **MRI:** is investigation of choice for Marrow, Soft tissues (Brain/ Spinal cord/Ligaments/Tendons/nerves/vessels) and Cartilage.

Basic Images in MRI are T_1 and T_2

- T_1 – 1st professional subject anatomy – so in T_1 image anatomy is seen.
- T_2 – 2nd professional subject pathology – so in T_2 image pathology is seen.

'Water is white on T_2'

Water is any body fluid example, synovial fluid/C.S.F/ inflammatory or traumatic edema.

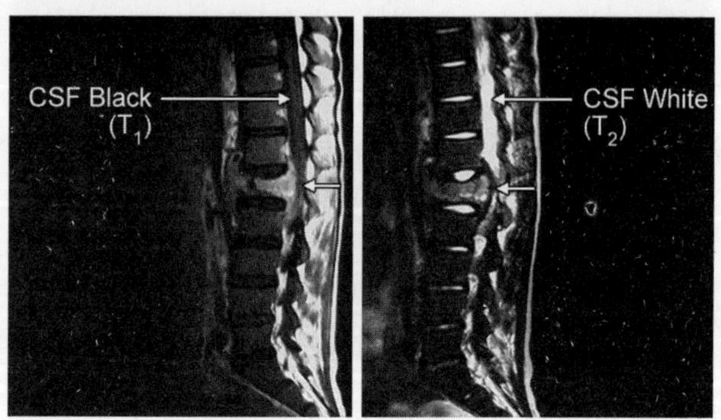

Fig. 1.6: MRI of spine (T_1 and T_2 images)

Please Note:

- Any occult fracture (not visualised on X-ray) e.g. Fracture neck femur ~ MRI is investigation of choice.
- Any fracture in which there is marrow edema example stress fracture- MRI is investigation of choice.
- Osteomyelitis starts in marrow of metaphysis—MRI is best radiological investigation.
- Tumors with marrow involvement, any micrometastasis or soft tissue component - MRI can aid in diagnosis.
- MRI is investigation of choice for Developmental Dysplasia of Hip (DDH).

D. **Bone scan:** can pick up - Blastic **(Osteoblastic)** activity - **Methylene diphosphonate** is taken up by osteoblasts on scanning the whole skeleton.

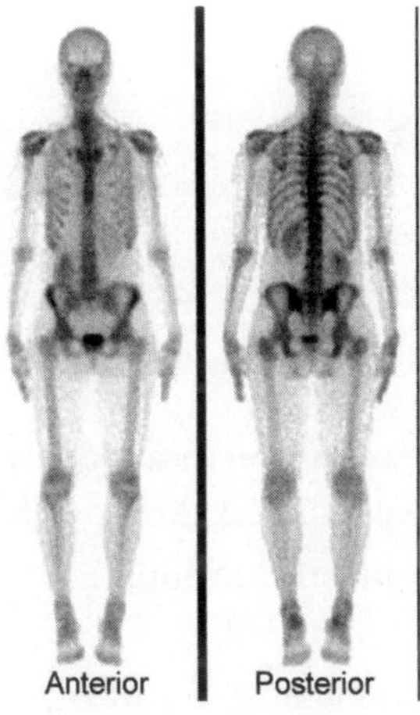

Fig. 1.7: Bone scan

Bone scan show activity in areas with increased osteoblastic activity example tumors, infection or fracture. Thus in cases with bilateral stress fractures bone scan is preferred investigation.

Note: investigation of choice for unilateral stress fracture is MRI and bilateral is Bone Scan.

It can pick up tumors that go from one bone to other i.e bone to bone metastasis. **BONE: B**one to bone/**O**steosarcoma/**N**euroblastoma/**E**wing sarcoma (maximum incidence).

Limitation: Bone Scan cannot indentify the source of unknown primary.

Note: Lesions with lytic activity do not show activity on bone scan e.g. multiple myeloma.

E. **PET CT:** Position emission tomography + CT Scan for whole body. It is a combination of 2 modalities.

18 F Deoxy glucose uptake by tumor cells (as they have anaerobic metabolism) and CT scan for all viscera so it can indentify unknown primary. (Bone Scan the uptake is by osteoblast and PET Scan by tumor cells).

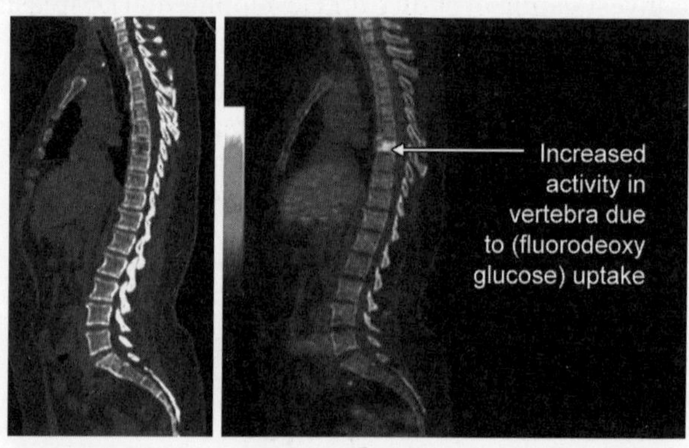

Fig. 1.8: PET scan

Thus PET-CT is more useful than Bone Scan as it can indentify primary and is more specific for tumor cells.

Limitation: Osteoblastic lesions have limited uptake where bone scan may be more valuable.

Remember that radiological diagnosis in cases of infection and tumors is suggestive never diagnostic.

F. Tumors and infection can mimic each other (clinically and radiologically) e.g. Osteosarcoma and Ewings sarcoma are two tumors that mimic osteomyelitis. (Both have accompanying pain, swelling, fever and increased local temperature).

Tumors and bone infections are usually metaphyseal and both need tissue diagnosis for differentiation.

- **Thus, Culture is gold standard for infection**
- **Histopathology is gold standard for tumors**

- So rule is Culture all biopsies, biopsy all cultures. That is whenever you obtain any sample from a suspected case of tumor or infection divide it into two parts send one for culture and other for histopathology.

Diagnostic is always tissue diagnosis.

Osteomyelitis

1. **X-ray:**

- Pyogenic Osteomyelitis on X-rays will show loss of soft tissue planes after 24-48 hours. (1st change)
- Day 7 to 10-solid periosteal reaction is identified. (1st Bony change)

Note:

- **In tuberculosis there is no periosteal reaction.**
- Chronic osteomyelitis- sclerosed dead bone (sequestrum) is important for diagnosis and onion peel appearance is the usual periosteal reaction.

2. **MRI:**

- MRI can pick up marrow changes in metaphysis. (Best radiological investigation for Oteomyelitis and Tuberculosis)

3. **Bone scan:**

- Bone scan is next in preference to MRI to pick up infections by picking osteoblastic activity at the site of infection.

4. Culture and growth of organism is most definitive diagnostic modality for Oteomyelitis.

Bone Tumors

1. X-ray is to localize the tumor.
2. CT scan is for extent and cortical lesion
3. MRI is for Marrow extent, micrometastasis and soft tissue involvement (Most preferred investigation for most tumors)
4. PET-CT and Bone scan for multiple lesions (PET-CT is better than Bone Scan)
5. Biopsy is definitive diagnostic modality for any tumor.

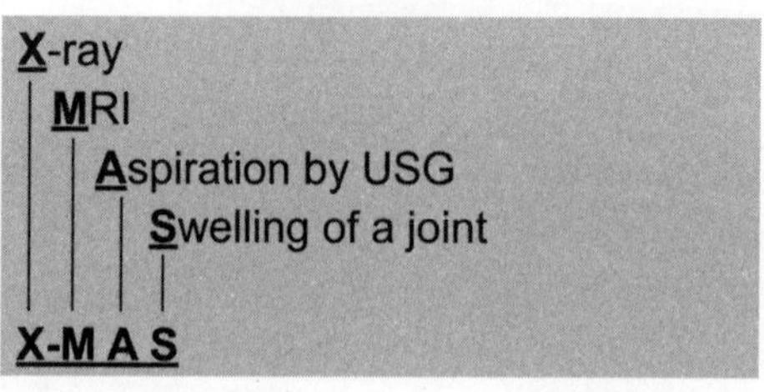

X-ray
MRI
Aspiration by USG
Swelling of a joint

X-M A S

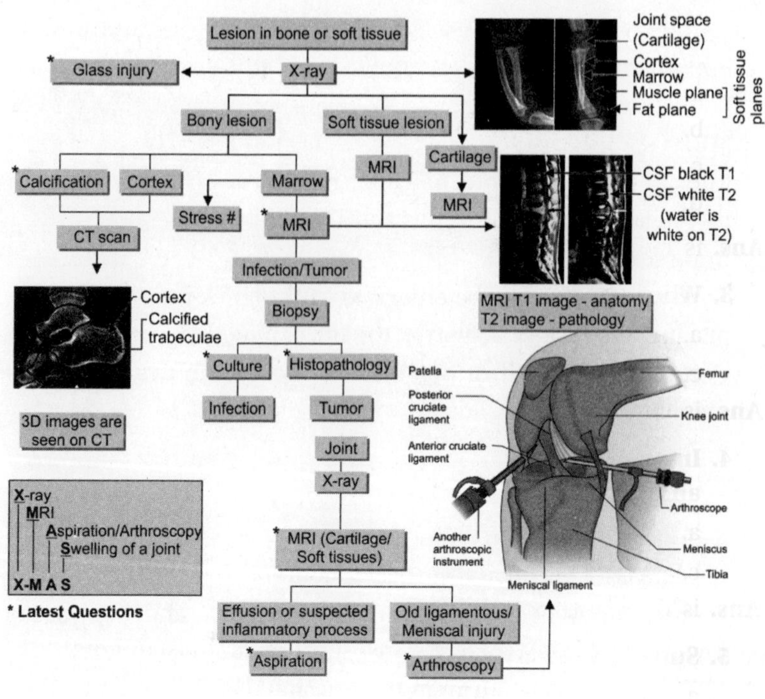

X-ray
MRI
Aspiration/Arthroscopy
Swelling of a joint

X-M A S

*** Latest Questions**

QUESTIONS

1. **"ORTHOPAEDICS" means:** *(Dec 2015)*
   a. Study of bone b. Study of fracture
   c. Straight child d. Study of disease of bone

Ans. is 'c' Straight child

2. **Identify the periosteal reaction:**

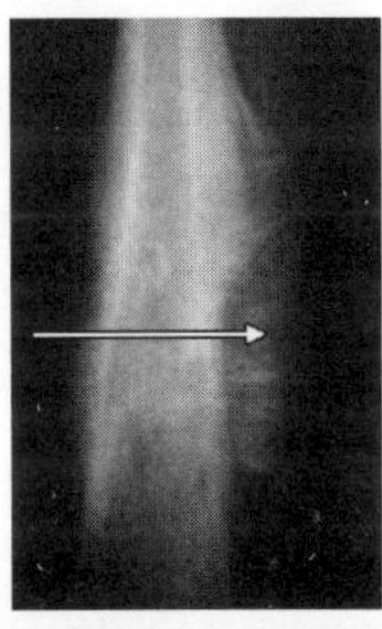

   a. Onion peel appearance
   b. Codman's triangle
   c. Sunburst appearance
   d. Onion ring appearance

Ans. is 'c' Sunburst appearance

3. **Who coined the term orthopaedics?** *(March 2010)*
   a. Louis Pasteur b. Edward Jenner
   c. Nicolas Andry d. Kuntscher

Ans. is 'c' Nicolas Andry

4. **Investigation of choice for congenital dislocation of hip in an infant is:**
   a. X-ray b. USG
   c. CT Scan d. MRI

Ans. is 'd' MRI

5. **Sunburst appearance seen in:**
   a. Osteosarcoma b. Osteopetrosis
   c. Osteomyelitis d. Osteo-radionecrosis

Ans. is 'a' Osteosarcoma

6. **Periosteal reaction in a case of acute osteomyelitis can be seen earliest at:** *(March 2012)*
   a. 5 days   b. 10 days
   c. 15 days   d. 20 days

Ans. is 'b' 10 days

7. **Radiological finding of Ewings sarcoma is:**
   a. Soap bubble appearance
   b. Sunray appearance
   c. Onion peel appearance
   d. Codman's triangle

Ans. is 'c' Onion peel appearance

Chapter 2

Infection of Bone and Joints

OSTEOMYELITIS

Acute Osteomyelitis

- Acute osteomyelitis is infection of bone.

Etiology

1. **Staphylococcus aureus is** the most common organism in all age groups
2. Post-traumatic osteomyelitis/ Post-surgical osteomyelitis - *S. aureus* (2012)
3. Immunocompromized (HIV) - *Staphylococcus aureus*
4. Salmonella is commonest organism in sickle cell anemia patients
5. *Pseudomonas aeruginosa* is commonest organism in Drug abusers
6. Human bite - *Eikenella corrodens*
7. Animal bite - *Pasteurella multocida*
8. Diabetic ulcer and Fight bites - Anaerobes

Pathology

- Most common mode of infection is **hematogenous**.
- In children **metaphysis** of long bone (usually **lower end femur** >upper end tibia) is earliest and most commonly involved site.
- In adults commonest site of infection is thoracolumbar spine.

Clinical Feature and Investigation

- Presenting complaints are Fever (>38.3°C), swelling of the limb, pain, systemic symptoms and increased levels of Total leucocyte counts, ESR and CRP. (Toxic child)

Note: Systemic signs are absent in immunocompromised and neonates.

- **Absent movements of a limb after ruling out trauma in pediatric population is osteomyelitis till proved otherwise.**

A. X-rays in <24 hours is normal

- 1st change on X-rays is loss of soft tissue planes. (>24–48 hours)
- 1st bony change is Periosteal reaction seen on day 7 to 10 (2nd week or day 10)- Solid Periosteal Reaction.
- Later features of bone destruction appear.

B. MRI is considered the best radiological investigation for bone infections because it can identify marrow edema (seen within 6 hours) and soft tissue extension in bone infections.

C. Tc99-MDP, Ga-67- citrate or Indium 111 labelled leucocytes (Best out of 3) are the 2nd best radiological investigation.

D. Gold standard is always tissue diagnosis (from the lesion) hence growth of organism on culture media is the best investigation for infections.

- Blood Culture is positive in 60% cases

Order in which investigations become positive is MRI-Bone scan-X-ray.

- Change of antibiotics or Surgery is considered if no improvement occurs within 48 hours of antibiotics

Subacute Osteomyelitis

Brodie's Abscess: Seen in immunocompetent Host!

- It is long standing localized pyogenic abscess in the bone (long standing because of strong defence mechanism of body)
- It usually involves long bones (metaphysis or diaphysis) e.g. Upper end tibia.
- Classical Brodie's abscess looks like a small walled off (Sclerotic margins) cavity in bone with little or no periosteal reaction.
- Usual isolated organism is *Staphylococcus aureus* (although most cultures are negative)

- Treatment: Trial of injectable antibiotics is given if it fails curettage of the cavity is carried out.

Chronic Osteomyelitis: "Usually a sequelae of inadequately treated acute osteomyelitis"

Causative organism; Staphylococcus aureus

1. *Sequestrum:* Avascular piece of bone surrounded by granulation tissue, it is pathognomic of chronic osteomyelitis.

It acts as nidus of infection and is most common cause of non healing sinus in chronic osteomyelitis.

2. Involucrum is dense sclerotic new bone surrounding the sequestrum formed from deep layers of stripped periosteum (usually obvious by the end of 2nd week).At least 2/3rd surface of sequestrum should be surrounded by involucrum before carrying out sequestrectomy (Removal of Sequestrum).
3. If infection persists, pus and tiny sequestrated spicules of bone may continue to discharge through perforations in involucrum (cloacae).
4. Cierney and Mader classification is used for chronic osteomyelitis

Treatment

1. Remove the sequestrum from Cavity or Saucerization of cavity (Leaving the Cavity Open)
2. Identify the organism and control the infection (most important step)
3. Fill the gap in Cavity with Bone graft/Bone cement (Poly Methyl MethAcrylate)
4. Provide a good soft tissue coverage- Local closure or by Myoplasty or Composite graft of Bone, Muscle and skin

SEPTIC ARTHRITIS

Septic (Pyogenic) Arthritis

Refers to Infection of Joint. Septic arthritis word is a misnomer as initially there is only infection of joint and if not treated early than Arthritis (Joint destruction) develops. Thus all sepsis of joints don't cause arthritis only inadequately treated ones do.

Etiology and Pathology

- The hematogenous route of infection is the most common route in all age groups

Epidemiology

- S. aureus – is the most common organism

(Absent movements of a joint after ruling out trauma in pediatric population is septic arthritis till proved otherwise.)

Diagnosis: X-rays are usually normal or may indicate soft tissue swellings, MRI may show effusion, synovitis or cartilage destruction and aspiration of joint will help to confirm the diagnosis by culture and sensitivity and can also help to differentiate from transient synovitis. Aspiration also decreases intra articular pressure and reduces chances of Avascular necrosis (AVN) of femoral head.

- Aspiration shows > 50,000 cells/l and > 75% Polymorphoneutrophils in septic arthritis.
- **Culture is the gold standard for diagnosis.**

Clinically

1. **Knee (most commonly affected joint)** – Position is Flexion
2. Hip-Position is Flexion, Abduction and External Rotation as this is the position of maximum capacity of joint to accommodate pus.

Treatment: **Arthrotomy** (opening the joint capsule), Surgical drainage (decompression) synovectomy **and antibiotics**. (2 weeks I/V and 4 weeks oral). Duration of antibiotics is same as osteomyelitis as usually focus is from the bone.

Note:

1. **Nonoperative treatment is not considered in joint infections as cartilage destruction occurs very rapidly and can cause permanent joint destruction.**
2. **Septic arthritis results in bony ankylosis and it is the most common cause of bony ankylosis.**

Ankylosis is the pathological fusion of bones in a joint.

Ankylosis may be:

1. **Fibrous ankylosis:** Two articular surfaces are fused by fibrous tissue. The features are:
   - Some movement of joint is possible (though just a jog of movement).

- Movements are painful.
- Most common cause is tubercular arthritis of hip and knee

2. **Bony ankylosis:** There is bony union between two articular surfaces. The features are : -
   - No movements possible.
   - Joint is painless
   - *Most common cause is acute suppurative arthritis (septic arthritis) > potts spine (T.B of Spine)*

Tom Smith Arthritis is septic arthritis of hip in infants which may **destroy the cartilaginous femoral head rapidly and completely (chondrolysis).** So child presents with limp, unstable gait, shortening of limb, telescopy and **increased hip movements** in all direction. Treatment includes procedures to stabilise the hip.

Tenosynovitis

It is infection within the flexor tendon sheath. Although the flexor sheath usually is involved, the radial and ulnar bursae may be involved as well.

Most common organism is S. aureus.

Kanavel signs are seen:

1. **Tenderness** over the involved sheath, (most significant)
2. Rigid positioning of the **finger in flexion,**
3. **Pain on attempts** to **hyperextend** the fingers, and
4. **Swelling of the involved part.**

When early tenosynovitis is suspected, immediate treatment with antibiotics and splinting may abort spread of the infection if the patient's symptoms have been present for less than 48 hours.

If drainage is required, an open or closed irrigation technique can be used. If an open technique is used, healing and rehabilitation are prolonged, and full motion may not be regained.

Felon or Whitlow

A felon is an abscess in the subcutaneous tissues of distal pulp of Most Commonly Thumb> index finger. The distal digital pulp is divided into tiny compartments by strong fibrous septa that traverse it from skin to bone. *S. aureus* is the organism most commonly isolated from fingertip infections.

Treatment consists of antibiotics **and longitudinal incision** for drainage.

Complications are Osteomyelitis >Tenosynovitis

Paronychia Most Common Infection of Hand

A paronychia ("runaround") infection usually is caused by the *S. aureus* into the soft-tissue fold around the fingernail (eponychium) associated with poor nail hygiene. It usually begins at one corner of the horny nail and travels under either the eponychium or the nail toward the opposite side. Treatment is incision and drainage and antibiotics.

QUESTIONS

1. **A 4-year-old child presented with limping and fever and has the given X-ray. Most likely diagnosis:** *(Recent Pattern Question 2017)*

   a. Osteomyelitis   b. Osteosarcoma
   c. Enchondroma   d. Aneurysmal bone cyst

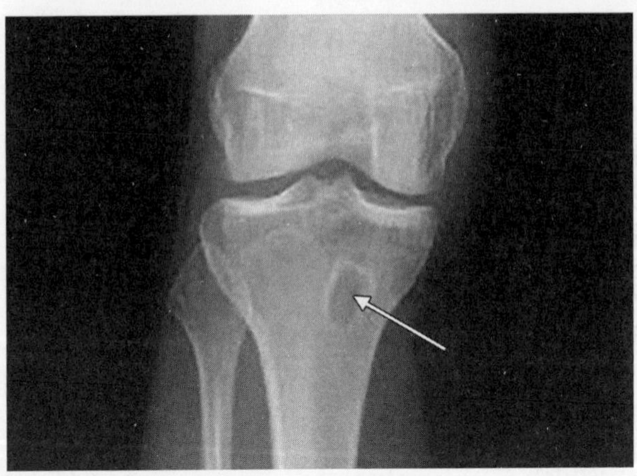

Ans. is 'a' Osteomyelitis

2. **Earliest X-ray finding in osteomyelitis:**

   a. Involucrum   b. Sequestrum
   c. Cloacae   d. Periosteal reaction

Ans. is 'd' Periosteal reaction

3. **Kanavel sign includes all EXCEPT:**
   a. Tenderness
   b. Flexion
   c. Pain upon passive flexion
   d. Uniform swelling

Ans. is 'c' Pain upon passive flexion

4. **Broadie's abscess, false statement:**
   a. Can be seen in Chronic osteomyelitis
   b. Can be seen in Subacute osteomyelitis
   c. Can be seen in Acute osteomyelitis
   d. Organism is staph. aureus

Ans. is 'c' Can be seen in Acute osteomyelitis

5. **Most common organism causing osteomyelitis:**
   a. Staph. aureus b. Strep. pneumonia
   c. H. influenza d. E. Coli

Ans. is 'a' Staph. aureus

6. **Most common site for Osteomyelitis**
   a. Epiphysis b. Metaphysis
   c. Diaphysis d. Sub-chondral growth plate

Ans. is 'b' Metaphysis

7. **Commonest cause of hematogenous osteomyelitis:**
   a. Streptococcus b. Staph. aureus
   c. Salmonella d. H. influenza

Ans. is 'b' Staph. aureus

8. **Brodie's abscess is seen in:**
   a. Acute osteomyelitis
   b. Chronic osteomyelitis
   c. Septic arthritis
   d. Subacute osteomyelitis

Ans. is 'd' Subacute osteomyelitis

9. **Bony ankylosis is noticed in case of**
   a. T.B arthritis b. Pyogenic arthritis
   c. Rheumatoid arthritis d. None

Ans. is 'b' Pyogenic arthritis

10. Purulent inflammation and infection of terminal pulp space of distal phalanges is known as:

a. Acute paronychium　b. Whitlow
c. Acute suppurative tenosynovitis
d. Apical subungual infection

Ans. is 'b' Whitlow

11. Acute Osteomyelitis is most commonly caused by: *(AI 02, UP 98)*

a. Staphylococcus aureus　b. Actinomyces bovis
c. Nocardia asteroids　d. Borrelia vincentii

Ans. is 'a' Staphylococcus aureus

12. The most common organism causing osteomyelitis in drug abusers is: *(PGI 97)*

a. E. coil　b. Pseudomonas
c. Klebsiella　d. Staph. aureus

Ans. is 'b' Pseudomonas

13. Chronic/recurrent paronychia is caused by:

a. Gram positive　b. Gram negative
c. Staphylococcus aureus　d. Fungal infection

Ans. is 'c' Staphylococcus aureus

14. Radiologically, earliest sign of osteomyelitis is:

a. Loss of muscle and fat planes *(DPG Feb. 09)*
b. Periosteal reaction
c. Callus formation　d. Presence of sequestrum

Ans. is 'a' Loss of muscle and fat planes

15. Cloacae are present in: *(NEET/DNB Pattern)*

a. Sequestrum　b. Involucrum
c. Normal bone　d. Myositis

Ans. is 'b' Involucrum

16. Sequestrum is best defined as: *(NEET/DNB Pattern)*

a. A piece of dead bone
b. A piece of dead bone surrounded by infected tissue
c. A piece of bone with poor vascularity
d. None

Ans. is 'b' A piece of dead bone surrounded by infected tissue

17. Commonest infection of hands is:

a. Acute paronychium
b. Terminals pulp space infection
c. Middle volar space infection
d. Apicals subungual infection

Ans. is 'a' Acute paronychium

18. Septic arthritis is diagnosed by: *(NEET/DNB Pattern)*

a. X-ray
b. Joint aspiration
c. USG
d. MRI

Ans. is 'b' Joint aspiration

19. Kanavel's sign is seen in: *(AIIMS Dec 07)*

a. Tenosynovitis
b. Trigger finger
c. Dupuytrens contracture
d. Carpal tunnel syndrome

Ans. is 'a' Tenosynovitis

20. Felon is *(NEET/DNB Pattern)*

a. Infection of nail fold
b. Infection of ulnar bursa
c. Infection of pulp space
d. Infection of DIP joint

Ans. is 'c' Infection of pulp space

21. Felon most common complication: *(NEET/DNB Pattern)*

a. Osteomyelitis
b. Subungual hematoma
c. Infective arthritis
d. None

Ans. is 'a' Osteomyelitis

22. In Bony ankylosis, there is: *(UP 98)*

a. Painless, No movement
b. Painful complete movement
c. Painless complete movement
d. Painful incomplete movement

Ans. is 'a' Painless, No movement

Chapter 3

Tuberculosis of Bone and Joints

- Tuberculosis has to Bone and Joints Hematogenous spread and Paucibacillary lesions
- Spine>hip>knee is the order of involvement of all musculoskeletal cases
- Spina Ventosa is Tuberculosis of short bones of hand.
- Tuberculosis of shoulder is dry (no effusion) - Caries sicca (dry)
- Pott's spine – Tuberculosis of spine
- Paradiscal region involvement is commonest, rarest is synovitis of facet joints, **Second Rarest is spinous process.**
- Most commonly affects Dorsolumbar area > Dorsal > lumbar > dorsolumbar junction
- 1st Neurological Sign: Increased deep tendon reflexes or Clonus,Twitching of muscles may be even earlier.

Investigations

- **X-ray:** Loss of Curvature of spine due to muscle spasm earliest sign>Paradiscal Lesion
- **MRI:** Best Radiological Investigation
- **CT Guided Biopsy:** or tissue diagnosis- Best Investigation

Treatment is Anti-Tubercular Therapy (ATT) + Surgery (if indicated)

Indication of Surgery

1. Bowel bladder involvement
2. Worsening on treatment
3. No improvement on treatment.

TUBERCULOSIS OF HIP STAGES

Stage 1: Synovitis-FABER-Flexion, abduction and external rotation.

Stage 2: Early arthritis- <1cm shortening + flexion, Adduction and internal rotation.

Stage 3: Late arthritis- > 1 cm shortening+ flexion, Adduction and internal rotation.

Stage 4: Wandering acetabulum-Femoral head is destroyed and wanders in acetabulum.

Stage 5: Fibrous ankylosis.

Note:

FABER at Hip: Flexion, Abduction and External Rotation

FADIR at Hip: Flexion, Adduction and Internal Rotation

TUBERCULOSIS OF KNEE

Triple deformity- Posterior subluxation, external rotation of leg and flexion of knee.

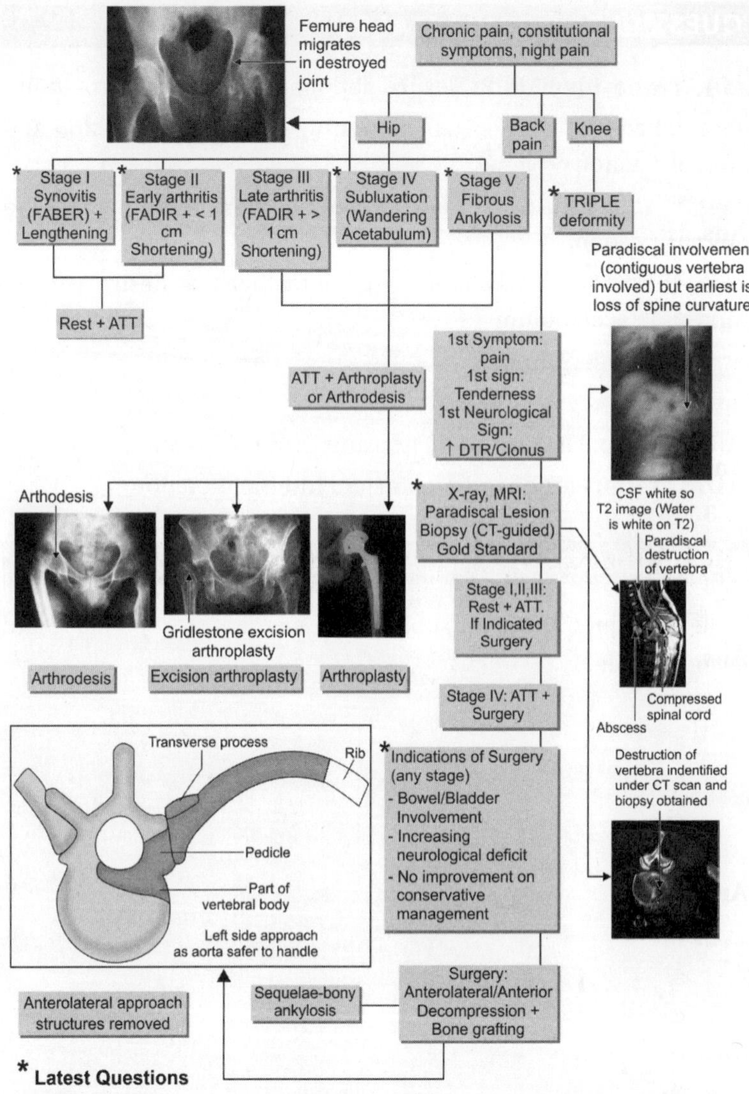

*** Latest Questions**

T.B hip and Knee sequelae is fibrous ankylosis and T.B spine there is bony ankylosis.
Arthrodesis: Surgical Fusion of Joint.

QUESTIONS

1. **Triple deformity is seen in all of the following conditions EXCEPT:** *(Recent Pattern Question 2017)*
   a. Knee TB
   b. Reactive arthritis
   c. Iliotibial contracture
   d. Poliomyelitis

Ans. is 'b' Reactive arthritis

2. **The spina ventosa is seen in:** *(Recent Pattern Question 2018)*
   a. Carpals
   b. Phalanges
   c. Dorsal spine
   d. Shoulder joint

Ans. is 'b' Phalanges

3. **Most common type of lesion in Pott's spine:** *(Recent Pattern Question 2018)*
   a. Central
   b. Anterior
   c. Paradiscal
   d. Appendiceal

Ans. is 'c' Paradiscal

4. **True about bony ankylosis:**
   a. Painful condition
   b. Tubercular arthritis is most common cause
   c. Septic arthritis leads to bony ankylosis
   d. Spine tuberculosis is the leading cause

Ans. is 'c' Septic arthritis leads to bony ankylosis

5. **Bony ankylosis is noticed in case of**
   a. TB arthritis
   b. Pyogenic arthritis
   c. Rheumatoid arthritis
   d. None

Ans. is 'b' Pyogenic arthritis

6. **Triple deformity of knee includes all EXCEPT:**
   a. Posterior subluxation of tibia
   b. Medial rotation of tibia
   c. Lateral rotation of tibia
   d. Flexion

Ans. is 'b' Medial rotation of tibia

7. Most common area involved of tubercular spine is:

a. Para-discal area

b. Central type

c. Anterior involvement

d. Appendicle involvement

Ans. is 'a' Para-discal area

8. What is the position of leg in tubercular hip in synovitis stage?

a. Flexion adduction internal rotation

b. Flexion abduction internal rotation

c. Flexion abduction external rotation

d. Extension abduction internal rotation

Ans. is 'c' Flexion abduction external rotation.

9. Spinaventosa is:

a. Tubercular dactylitis

b. TB of spine

c. TB of vertebral pedicles

d. Extra-axial TB

Ans. is 'a' Tubercular dactylitis

10. Commonest site for tuberculosis of the skeletal system is:

a. Hip
b. Knee

c. Ankle
d. Spine

Ans. is 'd' Spine

11. Tuberculosis in Pott's disease involves:

a. Hip Joint
b. Knee Joint

c. Spine
d. Wrist Joint

Ans. is 'c' Spine

12. In spinal tuberculosis, the commonest route of spread is:

a. Direct spread
b. Blood

c. Lymphatics
d. All of the above

Ans. is 'b' Blood

13. Commonest presenting symptom of Pott's spine is:

a. Cold abscess
b. Back pain
c. Decreased spinal movements
d. Collapse of spine

Ans. is 'b' Back pain

Commonest presenting symptom of Tuberculosis of spine (Potts spine) is back pain and sign is tenderness.

14. Night cries is a clinical feature of:

a. Oesteomyelitis b. Brucellosis
c. T.B d. Septic arthritis

Ans. is 'c' T.B.

15. Earliest sign in X-ray in TB spine is: *(March 2011)*

a. Paravertebral shadow b. Narrowing of disc space
c. Gibbus d. Straightening of spinal curves

Ans. is 'd' Straightening of spinal curves

16. Monoarticular joint involvement is seen in which of the following:

a. Primary osteoarthritis b. Rheumatoid arthritis
c. Tubercular arthritis d. Sero-neagtive spond-arthritis

Ans. is 'c' Tubercular arthritis

Tuberculosis is the most common cause of monoarticular arthritis.

17. Triple deformity of the knee is a complication of: *(September 2012)*

a. Tuberculosis b. Osteoarthritis
c. Septic arthritis d. All of the above

Ans. is 'a' Tuberculosis

18. Triple deformity in tubercular arthritis of the knee is:

a. Flexion, posterior subluxation and external rotation
b. Flexion, posterior subluxation and internal rotation
c. Extension, anterior subluxation and external rotation
d. Extension, anterior subluxation and internal rotation

Ans. is 'a' Flexion, posterior subluxation and external rotation.

19. Caries sicca is the characteristic feature of:

a. Tuberculosis of shoulder joint
b. Avascular necrosis of head of humerus
c. Osteoarthritis of shoulder
d. Frozen shoulder

Ans. is 'a' Tuberculosis of shoulder joint.

20. The most common sequelae of tuberculous spondylitis is:

a. Fibrous ankylosis
b. Bony ankylosis
c. Pathological dislocation
d. Chronic osteomyelitis

Ans. is 'b' Bony ankylosis

21. Fibrous ankylosis is caused by which of the following:

a. Septic arthritis
b. TB arthritis
c. Behcet's disease
d. Psoriatic arthritis

Ans. is 'b' TB arthritis

22. Pott's spine is commonest in spine: *(DELHI 94)*

a. Cervical
b. Thoracic
c. Lumbar spine
d. Sacral

Ans. is 'b' Thoracic

23. The most common sequelae of tuberculous spondylitis in an adolescent is: *(AI 05, NEET/DNB Pattern)*

a. Fibrous ankylosis
b. Bony-ankylosis
c. Pathological dislocation
d. Chronic osteomyelitis

Ans. is 'b' Bony-ankylosis

24. A 35-year-old lady with chronic backache. On X-ray she had a D12 collapse. But Intervertebral disc space is maintained. All are possible except: *(AIIMS Nov 10)*

a. Multiple myeloma
b. Osteoporosis
c. Metastasis
d. Tuberculosis

Ans. is 'd' Tuberculosis

25. The early feature of Pott's paraplegia Is: *(DPG 10)*

a. Flexor spasm
b. Increased tendon jerk
c. Ankle clonus
d. Sensory loss

Ans. is 'b' Increased tendon jerk

26. False about Pott's spine: *(NEET/DNB Pattern)*

a. Commonest at dorsolumbar junction
b. Always heals by chemotherapy
c. Back pain is an early symptom
d. There is disc space narrowing on X-ray

Ans. is 'b' Always heals by chemotherapy

Chapter 4

Orthopedics Oncology

MOST COMMON SITE OF PRIMARY BONE TUMORS

A. Epiphyseal

- **Chondroblastoma (before physeal closure)-purely epiphyseal**
- Osteoclastoma/Giant cell tumor (after physeal closure in adults).

B. Metaphyseal (Most Common Site for Bone Tumors)

- Enchondroma
- Bone cyst
- Osteosarcoma
- Osteoclastoma (in children)

Note: Osteomyelitis also starts in metaphysis

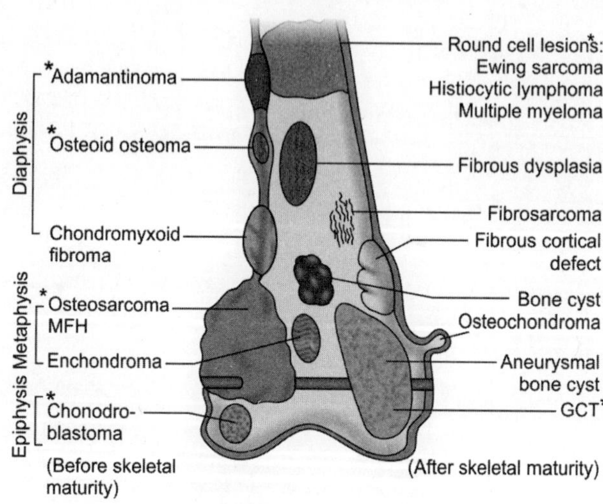

Fig. 4.1: Sites of bone tumors

Diaphyseal

1. Round cell lesions -**Ewing's sarcoma**
2. Lymphoma
3. Multiple myeloma
4. Admantinoma
5. Osteoid osteoma

Most Common Sites

Unicameral bone cyst	Upper end Humerus
Aneurysmal bone cyst	**Lower limb metaphysis (Tibia and femur)**
Osteochondroma	Distal femur
Osteoid osteoma	Femur >Tibia
Osteoblastoma	Vertebrae
Osteoma (Ivory or Compact or Eburnated)	Skull and facial bones
Enchondroma	Short bones of hand
Chordoma	Sacrum (most common) > sphenooccipital region (clivus)> anterior vertebral body, i.e. involves only axial skeleton
Adamantinoma (Long bone)	Tibia
Ameloblastoma	Mandible
Osteoclastoma (GCT)	Lower end of Femur
Fibrous dysplasia	**Upper femur monostotic (commoner) Craniofacial region – Polyostotic**
Multiple myeloma	Lumbar vertebrae
Osteosarcoma	Lower end of femur
Ewing's sarcoma	Femur
Chondrosarcoma	Pelvis
Secondary tumors	Dorsal vertebrae (Secondaries in bone are commonest from Breast > prostate > lung > kidney)

AGE PREDILECTION

1st decade:

(i) Ewings sarcoma (5-20 years)
(ii) Unicameral bone cyst

2nd decade:

(i) Osteosarcoma
(ii) Aneurysmal bone cyst

After Skeletal Maturity (20-40 years)

GCT

> 40 years of age

(i) Metastases—Most common bone tumor
(ii) Multiple myeloma—Most common primary bone tumor

Note: Ewings sarcoma is commonest Bone tumor of 1st decade but its peak incidence is 2nd decade. (2012)

Remember

1st decade Diaphyseal bone tumor -Ewings sarcoma
2nd decade Metaphyseal bone tumor -Osteosarcoma

Classical Radiological Features*

• Sun ray appearance*/ Codman's triangle	Osteosarcoma but can be seen in any malignant lesion
• Onion peel appearance*	Ewing sarcoma but can be seen in any malignant lesion or chronic osteomyelitis
• Soap bubble appearance*	**Osteoclastoma (GCT)** > adamantinoma
• Patchy calcification*	Chondrogenic tumors (Chondrosarcoma > Chondroblastoma)
• Homogenous calcification	Osteogenic tumors (Osteosarcoma)

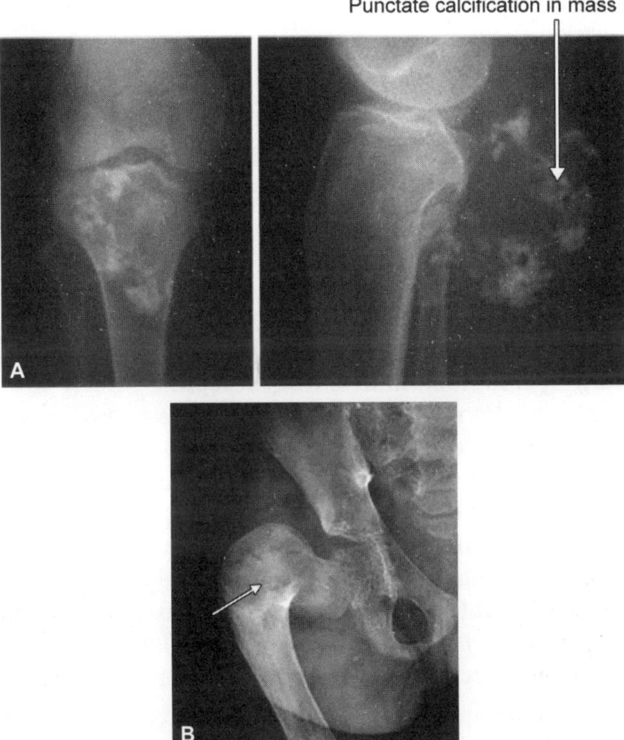

Figs. 4.2A to C: (A) Patchy calcification; (B) Shepherd crook deformity; (C) Homogenous calcification.

Order of investigations usually X-rays than MRI and then biopsy.

Biopsy is the ultimate diagnostic technique for bone tumors.

Enneking's classification system is used for bone tumors.

Treatment

The goal of treatment in a patient with a primary malignancy of the musculoskeletal system is to make the patient disease free. The goal of treatment of a patient with metastatic carcinoma to bone is to minimize pain and to preserve function. The optimal treatment of the tumor often requires a combination of radiation therapy, chemotherapy, and surgery.

Radiation Therapy

Most primary bone malignancies are relatively radio resistant. Exceptions are the **marrow cell tumors, including multiple myeloma, lymphoma, and Ewing sarcoma, which are each exquisitely sensitive. Carcinomas metastatic to bone, with the exception of renal cell carcinoma, also frequently are sensitive to radiation treatment.** Most radiation treatment protocols deliver 150 to 200 cGy/d until the target dose is achieved. This dose ranges from **30 to 40 Gy for myeloma to 60 Gy for treatment of a soft-tissue sarcoma. Radiotherapy is rarely used for benign conditions. (Possible exceptions include an extensive pigmented villonodular synovitis that cannot be controlled by surgery or a large spinal giant cell tumor.)**

Radiation therapy is associated with significant acute and long-term complications. Acutely, the most common complication is skin irritation. Other common acute side effects include gastrointestinal upset, urinary frequency, fatigue, anorexia, and extremity edema. Late effects include chronic edema, fibrosis, osteonecrosis, and pathological fracture. Malignant transformation of irradiated tissues (i.e., radiation sarcoma) is being reported with increasing frequency in survivors of childhood and adolescent cancers. These secondary sarcomas occur with a mean lag time of approximately 10 years and often are associated with a poor prognosis. Most common type is osteosarcoma.

Chemotherapy

Adjuvant chemotherapy refers to chemotherapy administered postoperatively to treat presumed micrometastases. Neoadjuvant chemotherapy refers to chemotherapy administered before surgical resection of the primary tumor. Preoperative chemotherapy frequently causes regression of the primary tumor, making a successful limb salvage (Preserving) operation easier. **Neoadjuvant**

chemotherapy followed by surgical resection allows for histological evaluation of the effectiveness of treatment. This is one of the most valuable prognostic indicators of successful long-term outcome. In addition, histological evaluation may lead to alteration of further chemotherapy in poor responders. Preoperative chemotherapy theoretically may decrease the spread of tumor cells at the time of surgery. On the same approach there is improvement in survival of osteosarcoma and the current 5-year survival rate for osteosarcoma is approximately 70%. In general, chemotherapy is not useful for cartilaginous lesions and most other low-grade malignancies.

Surgical Therapy

In orthopaedic oncology, the surgical margin is described by one of four terms—intralesional, marginal, wide, or radical. Amputations and limb-sparing resections may be associated with any of the four types of margins, and the margin must be specifically defined with each procedure.

Intralesional - Enters tumor leaving gross residual tumor within the bed.

Marginal - Plane through reactive zone around tumor.

Wide local excision (Most commonly used) cuff of normal tissue completely encircling, the tumor is taken out. (Usual cuff of normal tissue is 3 cm)

Radical or amputation - Tissue from joint to joint and muscle from origin to insertion is excised.

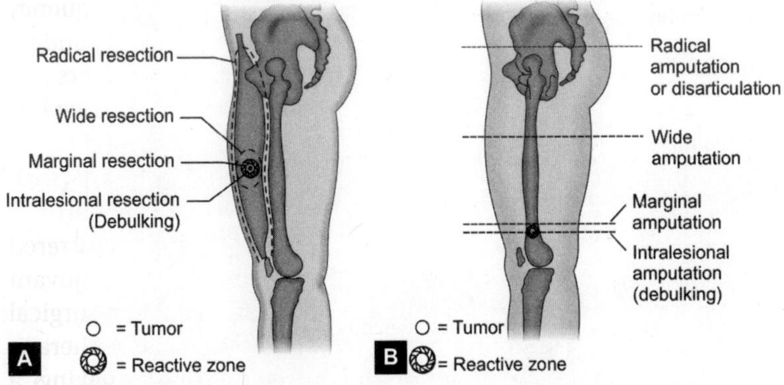

Figs. 4.3A and B: (A) Enneking's margins for tumor excision; (B) Enneking's margins for amputation

Curettage is removing or curetting or scooping out the contents of the lesion e.g. for simple bone cyst. If to it additional chemical (Phenol/Poly Methy Meth Acrylate/Liquid Nitrogen/hydrogen peroxide/Argon beam laser) is added to kill the residual cells to decrease the rate for recurrence it is called as extended curettage. Extended curettage is used for GCT, Enchondroma and Aneurysmal bone cyst. Least rate of recurrence in extended curettage is seen with Liquid Nitrogen.

Note: Most of the benign tumors and cartilaginous tumors are treated by surgery.

Osteosarcoma and cartilaginous tumors are radioresistant.

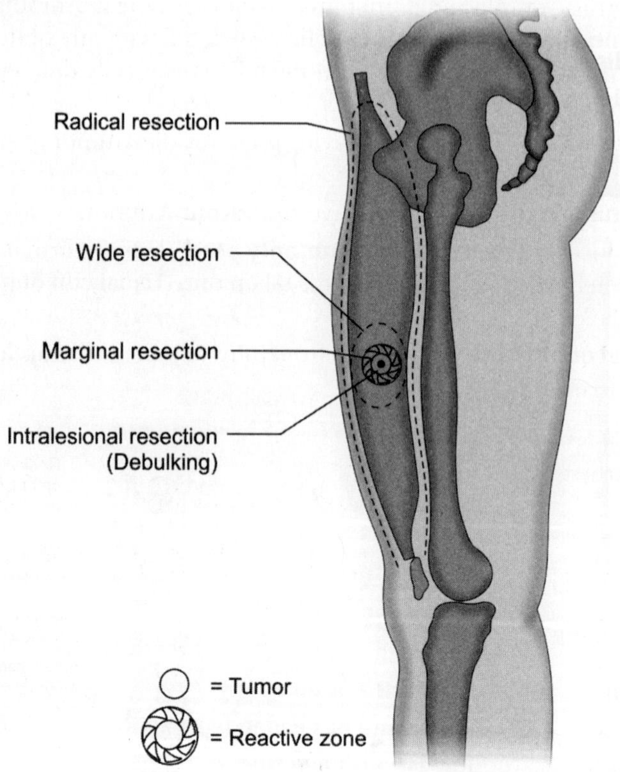

Fig. 4.4: Ennekings margins for tumor excision

Important Points to Remember

- Most common bone tumors - Secondaries.
- Most common primary malignant bone tumor - Multiple Myeloma.
- Second most common primary malignant bone tumor - Osteosarcoma.
- Commonest malignant bone tumor of flat bone - Chondrosarcoma.
- **Commonest tumor of skull vault-ivory Osteoma or compact osteoma or eburnated osteoma.**
- Commonest true benign tumor - Osteoid osteoma.
- Most common benign tumor of spine - Hemangioma.
- **Benign bone tumor** have well defined margin, uniform consistency on feel and narrow zone of activity.
- **Malignant tumor have ill-defined margins, variable consistency and wide zone of activity.**

BENIGN BONE TUMORS

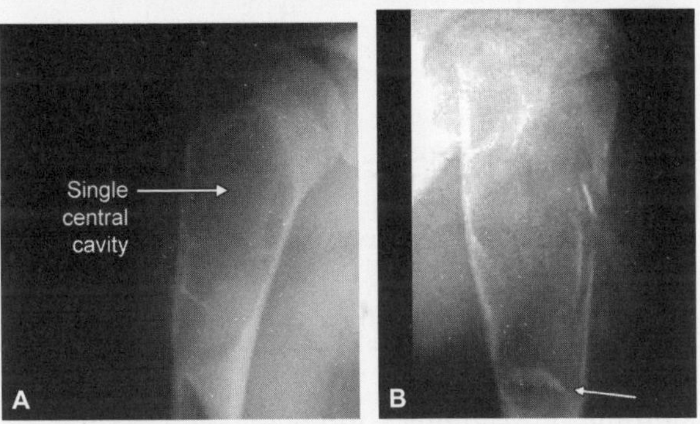

Figs. 4.5A and B: (A) Unicameral or simple bone cyst; (B) Fallen fragment (leaf) sign

Unicameral bone cyst: is seen at upper end of humerus it has single cavity, Central cyst and has Fallen leaf sign or Trap door sign. The treatment option is curettage and bone grafting, Steroid or Sclerosant injection. Radiotherapy is not used.

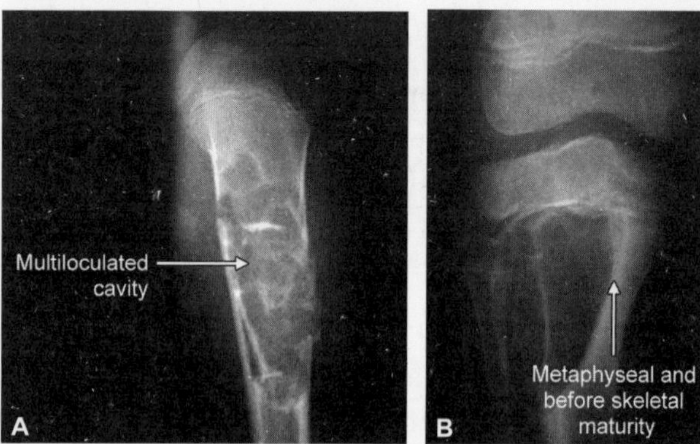

Figs. 4.6A and B: Aneurysmal bone cyst

Aneurysmal Bone cyst: is seen in lower limbs (Tibia) Eccentric cavity, Multiloculated. It is seen before skeletal maturity. Treatment is extended curettage.

Osteochondroma – Bony Growth with Cartilage Cap

- **Treatment:** Extraperiosteal resection(Removal along with periosteum).

Osteoid Osteoma – M.C. Femur Diaphysis

- It is commonest benign true bone tumor, exceeded in incidence only by osteochondroma and nonossifying fibroma.
- The typical patient with an osteoid osteoma has pain that is worse at night and is relieved by aspirin or other nonsteroidal antiinflammatory medications.
- CT is the best study to identify the nidus and confirm the diagnosis.
- Surgical management involves removal of the entire nidus burr-downtechnique.
- Radiofrequency ablation the preferred modality.

Enchondroma

- Enchondroma-most common tumor of bones of hand.
- Multiple enchondromatosis is also known as Ollier disease.
- Maffuccis syndrome is Enchondroma, subcutaneous hemangioma and phlebolith.
- Treatment is extended Curettage

Chondroblastoma/Codman's Tumor-Epiphyseal bone tumor

Classic **"chicken wire"** calcification

Giant Cell Tumor: Epiphyseal

Tumor of lower end of radius is GCT fill proved otherwise.

GCT has 2 types of cells giant cells and mononuclear cells (Malignant cells).

Radiologically GCT is the only tumor which can go very close to the joint surface.

Most common site is Distal Femur

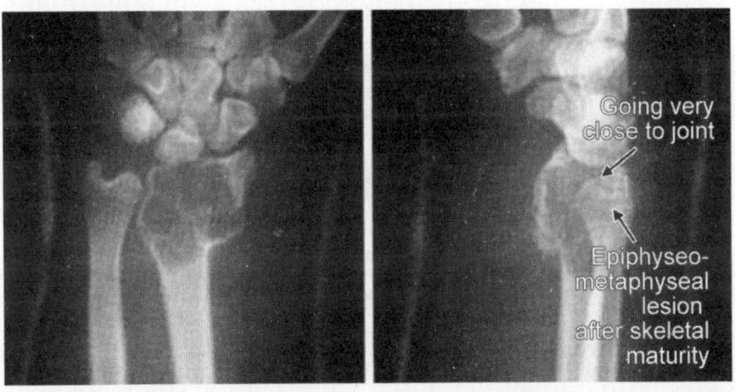

Fig 4.7: Giant cell tumor of lower end radius

Treatment of Osteoclastoma (GCT)

1. Extended Curettage by PMMA or phenol or liquid nitrogen and bone grafting
   It is procedure of choice for most lesions.
2. Excision
   Lower end of ulna
   Upper end of fibula
3. Excision and replacement by vascularized bone graft
   Lower end of radius where upper end of fibula is grafted

Giant Cell Variants (Tumor with Giant Cells)

- Brown tumor of hyperparathyroidism
- Aneurysmal bone cyst (closest) and unicameral bone cyst
- Non-ossifying fibroma (commonest) and fibrous dysplasia
- Osteoblastoma and osteosarcoma
- Chondromyxoid fibroma and Chondroblastoma

Adamantinoma: Most common long bone affected Tibia.

Ameloblastoma most commonly affects mandible.

Please note that **most common tumor of mandible is squamous cell carcinoma.**

Fibrous Dysplasia

- McCune-Albright syndrome refers to polyostotic fibrous dysplasia, cutaneous pigmentation (café au lait spots), and endocrine abnormalities. (Precocious puberty).
- Mazabraud syndrome is polyostotic fibrous dysplasia with intra-muscular myxomas.
- Fibrous dysplasia of proximal femur has shepherd crook deformity

MALIGNANT BONE TUMORS

Osteosarcoma

- Osteosarcoma may be more common in patients with the hereditary form of retinoblastoma and Li-Fraumeni syndrome.
- Osteosarcoma is the most common radiation induced sarcoma.
- **Osteosarcoma is radioresistant.**
- **Osteosarcoma is a pulsatile bone tumor.**
- Chemotherapy + Limb Salvage Surgery + Chemotherapy (Methotrexate is most important).
- Etoposide is not included in the 'T-10'protocol for osteosarcoma.

Ewings sarcoma - Presentation is like osteomyelitis

Classically, Ewing sarcoma appears radiographically as a destructive lesion in the diaphysis of a long bone (Femur) with an "onion skin" periosteal reaction.

Origin is from marrow cells and it is a round cell tumor.

The t(11; 22) (q24; q12) is the most common translocation of Ewing sarcoma and is present in greater than 90% of cases.

MIC 2 (CD 99) positive cells, glycogen positive cells **are seen in Biopsy.**

Poor prognositc Factors are: Males age > 12, Fever, anemia, Increased TLC, platelets, LDH, Proximal lesion, **chemoresistance, relapse and distant metastasis. (Last 3 are worst prognostic factors).**

Treatment of Ewing's Sarcoma – Chemotherapy followed by surgery followed by chemotherapy.

ABCD (Actinomycin D/Bleomycin/Cyclophosphamide/Doxorubicin) is chemotherapy

---

Chondrosarcoma is most common tumor associated with Hyperglycemia.

Treatment of Chondrosarcoma is surgical excision.

Chordoma

Chordoma is rare malignant tumor originating from the remnants of primitive notochord. Physaliphorous cells are seen. It commonly occurs in the sacrococcygeal or in the spheno-occipital regions. Sacrum is the most common site.

Multiple Myeloma

Multiple myeloma is tumor of plasma cells.

Elderly patient with bone pains, increased ESR and hypercalcemia diagnosis is multiple myeloma till proved otherwise.

Punched out lytic lesions are seen on skull.

Metastatic Bone Disease

- Most common primary is Breast>Prostate >Lung overall
- Most common sites of primary for bone metastasis.
  - In males – Prostate > Lung
  - In Female – Breast > Lung
  - In Children – Neuroblastoma
- Skeletal sites most frequently involved
  - Spine (Dorsal)
- Purely Osteoblastic secondaries
  - Prostate

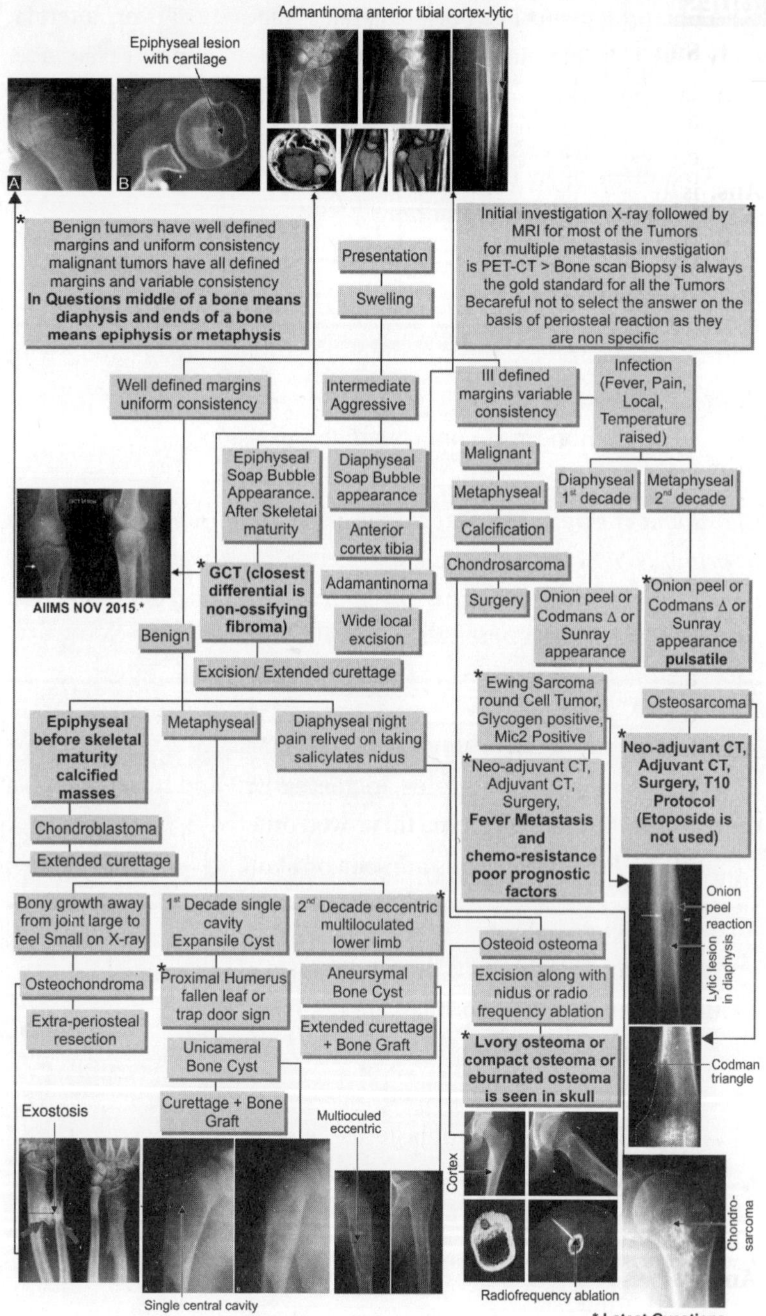

* Latest Questions

QUESTIONS

1. Sunray appearance in osteosarcoma is due to:

(Recent Pattern Question 2018)

a. Bone destruction b. Periosteal reaction

c. Vascular calcification d. Bone hypertrophy

Ans. is 'b' Periosteal reaction

2. A child with pain in lower limb presented with this X-ray. Which is the probable diagnosis?

(Recent Pattern Question 2017)

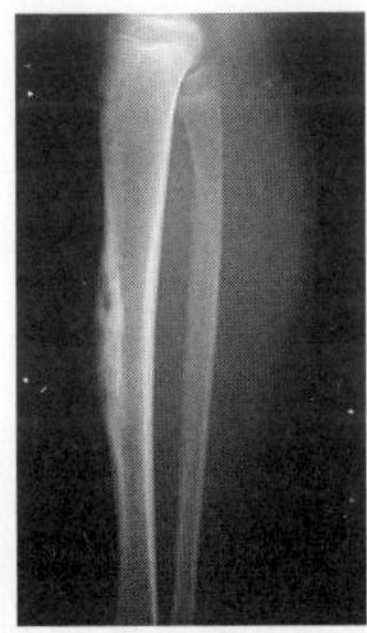

a. Osteosarcoma b. Osteoid osteoma

c. Ewing's sarcoma d. Osteofibrous dysplasia

Ans. is 'd' Osteofibrous dysplasia

3. Diagnosis is:

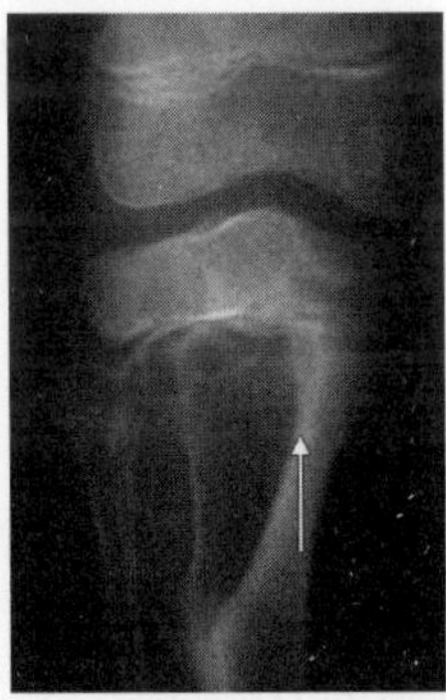

a. Unicameral bone cyst b. Aneurysmal bone cyst

c. Giant Cell tumor d. Osteosarcoma

Ans. is 'b' Aneurysmal bone cyst

4. Which of the following is an epiphyseal tumor?

(Recent Pattern Question 2017)

a. Osteoid osteoma b. Adamantinoma

c. Osteosarcoma d. Chrondroblastoma

Ans. is 'd' Chrondroblastoma

5. Sunburst appearance usually seen in:

a. Osteosarcoma b. Osteopetrosis

c. Osteomyelitis d. Osteoradionecrosis

Ans. is 'a' Osteosarcoma

6. X-ray wrist showing soap bubble appearance in epiphyseal region. Diagnosis:

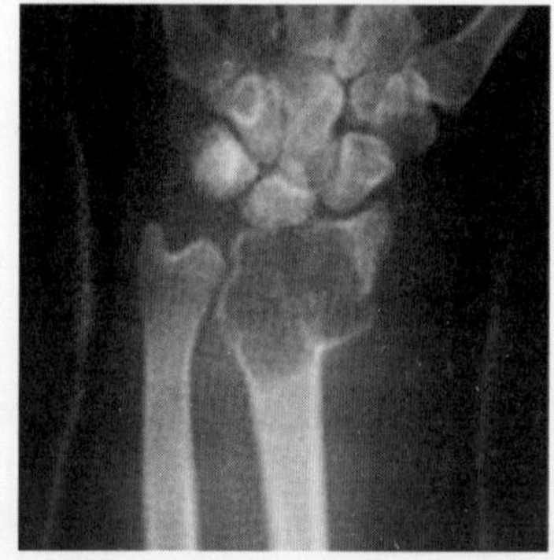

a. Giant cell tumor b. Osteosarcoma

c. Osteochondroma d. Osteoid osteoma

Ans. is 'a' Giant cell tumor

7. True about osteosarcoma:

a. Very radio sensitive tumor

b. Sunburst appearance exclusively found here

c. Most commonly seen in diaphyseal area

d. Tissue biopsy is investigation of choice

Ans. is 'd' Tissue biopsy is investigation of choice

8. Fallen leaf sign is seen in?

a. Aneurysmal bone cyst b. Simple bone cyst

c. Osteosarcoma d. Osteoclastoma

Ans. is 'b' Simple bone cyst

9. Aspirin is useful in which type of bone tumor?

a. Osteonecrosis b. Osteopetrosis

c. Osteoid osteoma d. Ewing sarcoma

Ans. is 'c' Osteoid sarcoma

10. Most common presenting age of Ewing's sarcoma is:

a. First decade b. Second decade

c. Third decade d. Fourth decade

Ans. is 'b' Second decade

11. The tumor which has a predilection for ephiphysis is:

a. Chondroblastoma b. Osteosarcoma

c. Osteochondroma d. Ewing's sarcoma

Ans. is 'a' Chondroblastoma

12. Which bone tumour arises from an area around epiphyseal plate:

a. Osteosarcoma b. Ewings sarcoma

c. Chondroblastoma d. Chondromyxoid fibroma

Ans. is 'c' Chondroblastoma

13. Bone tumour arising from metaphysis: *(September 2012)*

a. Osteogenic sarcoma b. Ewing sarcoma

c. Osteoclastoma d. Osteoid osteoma

Ans. is 'a' Osteogenic sarcoma

14. Osteosarcoma commonly affects:

a. Metaphysis b. Diaphysis

c. Epiphysis d. None of the above

Ans. is 'a' Metaphysis

15. The most common bone sarcoma in children is:

a. Ewing's sarcoma b. Fibrosarcoma

c. Chondrosarcoma d. Osteosarcoma

Ans. is 'a' Ewing's sarcoma

16. Bone forming tumors are all except:

a. Osteoid osteoma b. Osteoblastoma

c. Osteochondroma d. Aggressive osteoblastoma

e. Osteosarcoma

Ans. is 'c' Osteochondroma

17. Which of the following is not a bone forming tumour?

a. Osteoma b. Osteoblastoma

c. Chondro-sarcoma d. Osteosarcoma

Ans. is 'c' Chondro-sarcoma

18. Shepherd Crook deformity is a feature of:

a. Fibrous dysplasia b. Post polio paralysis

a. Cerebral palsy c. Perthe's disease

Ans. is 'a' Fibrous dysplasia

19. Soap bubble appearance is a classical X-ray finding in:

a. Giant cell tumor of bone

b. Osteosarcoma

c. Reticulum cell sarcoma

d. Adamantinoma

Ans. is 'a' Giant cell tumor of bone

20. Mottled calcification with in the tumor is seen in X-ray is:

a. Osteosarcoma b. Ewing's tumor

c. Osteoclastoma d. Chondrosarcoma

Ans. is 'd' Chondrosarcoma

21. Sunray appearance on X-ray may be seen in:

(September 2008, March 2013 (c)

a. Osteoclastoma b. Osteoblastoma

c. Osteosarcoma d. Chondroblastoma

Ans. is 'c' Osteosarcoma

22. Radiological finding of ewings sarcoma is:

a. Soap bubble appearance

b. Sunray appearance

c. Onion peel appearance

d. Codman's triangle

Ans. is 'c' Onion peel appearance

23. Solitary bone cyst is most common in the

a. Upper end of humerus

b. Lower end of humerus

c. Upper end of fibula

d. Lower end of femur

Ans. is 'a' Upper end of humerus

24. Commonest location of aneurysmal bone cyst is:

a. Femur
b. Pelvis
c. Vertebrae
d. Tibia

Ans. is 'd' Tibia

25. MC cause of pathological fracture in a child is:

a. Malignancy
b. Bone cyst
c. Fibrous dysplasia
d. Paget's disease

Ans. is 'b' Bone cyst

26. Following are seen in fibrous dysplasia EXCEPT:

(September 2004)

a. Café-au-lait spots
b. No premalignant change
c. Expanding rib lesions
d. Expanding lesions of maxilla

Ans. is 'b' No premalignant change

27. A patient is having diagnosed as GCT in upper end of fibula. Treatment of this is:

a. Excision © Turn-o-plasty
b. Excision © fibular graft
c. Excision
d. Chemotherapy

Ans. is 'c' Excision

28. Adamantinoma is a common tumour of:

a. Mastoid bones
b. Skull bones
c. Jaw bones
d. Lower end of tibia
e. Femur bone

Ans. is 'd' Lower end of tibia

29. An intramedullary tumour occurring in the lower metaphysis of the tibia in a 15 year old male is most likely to be:

a. Ewing's sarcoma
b. Giant cell tumour
c. Chondrosarcoma
d. Osteosarcoma

Ans. is 'd' Osteosarcoma

30. Tumour which can occur following exposure to radiation is:

a. Osteosarcoma
b. Osteoblastoma
c. Ewing's sarcoma
d. Osteoclastoma

Ans. is 'a' Osteosarcoma

31. Most common primary bone tumour in adult bone is: *(March 2011)*

a. Chondrosarcoma b. Osteogenic sarcoma
c. Adamantinoma d. Ewings sarcoma

Ans. is 'b' Osteogenic sarcoma

32. Treatment of Ewing's tumour:

a. Local ablation + chemotherapy
b. Excision of tumour + Chemotherapy
c. Local ablation + Radiotherapy
d. Only Radiotherapy

Ans. is 'b' Excision of tumor + Chemotherapy

33. Common sites of Chondrosarcoma is:

a. Lower end of femur & upper end of tibia.
b. Femur, tibia, flat bones
c. Flat bones and upper ends of femur
d. Lower femur, upper tibia and lower radius.

Ans. is 'c' Flat bones and upper ends of femur

34. Physaliphorous cell (Larger vacuolated cells) on histopathology are characteristic of:

a. Osteosarcoma b. Osteoclastoma
c. Chordoma d. Chondrosarcoma

Ans. is 'c' Chordoma

35. Which of the following is seen in multiple myeloma:

a. Raised serum calcium b. Decreased serum calcium
c. Normal serum calcium d. None of the above

Ans. is 'a' Raised serum calcium

36. Punched out lesion in the skull is indicative of:

a. Ewings sarcoma b. Multiple myeloma
c. Metastasis d. Osteosarcoma

Ans. is 'b' Multiple myeloma

37. Most common tumor of spine is:

a. Secondaries b. Ewings sarcoma
c. Osteosarcoma d. Multiple myeloma

Ans. is 'a' Secondaries

38. MC malignant bone tumour is: *(September 2003)*

a. Osteosarcoma b. Osteoclastoma

c. Secondaries d. Multiple myeloma

Ans. is 'c' Secondaries

39. Osteoblastic secondaries arises from: March 2003

a. Renal carcinoma b. Thyroid carcinoma

c. GIT carcinoma d. Prostate carcinoma

Ans. is 'd' Prostate carcinoma

40. Metastatic tumour causing spinal cord compression are all EXCEPT: *(March 2004)*

a. Lung carcinoma b. Breast carcinoma

c. Lymphoma d. Meningioma

Ans. is 'd' Meningioma

41. According to a newer hypothesis Ewings sarcoma arises from: *(AI 99)*

a. Epiphysis b. Diaphysis

c. Medullary cavity d. Cortex

Ans. is 'c' Medullary cavity

42. Classification system of bone tumors is:

a. Enneking b. Manchester

c. Edmonton d. TNM

Ans. is 'a' Enneking

43. Which of the following occurs in epiphysis: *(PGI Dec 01)*

a. Osteoclastoma b. Chondroblastoma

c. Osteochondroma d. Ewing's sarcoma

Ans. is 'b' Chondroblastoma

44. Babu a 19 yrs old male has a small circumscribed sclerotic swelling over diaphysis of femur; likely diagnosis is: *(AI 01, AIIMS Nov 01)*

a. Osteoclastoma b. Osteosarcoma

c. Ewing sarcoma d. Osteoid osteoma

Ans. is 'd' Osteoid osteoma

45. Most common bone tumor in hand: *(AIIMS June 97)*

a. Exostosis b. Giant cell tumor

c. Enchondroma d. Synovial sarcoma

Ans. is 'c' Enchondroma

46. Soap bubble appearance at lower end of radius, the treatment of choice is: *(AIIMS June 98)*

a. Local excision

b. Excision and bone grafting

c. Amputation

d. Radiotherapy

Ans. is 'b' Excision and bone grafting

47. Most common site of osteogenic sarcoma: *(AI 01, AIIMS June 2K)*

a. Femur, upper end b. Femur, lower end

c. Tibia, upper d. Tibia, lower end

Ans. is 'b' Femur, lower end

48. X-ray appearance of osteosarcoma are all except: *(NEET/DNB Pattern)*

a. Periosteal reaction b. Codman's triangle

c. Soap-bubble d. Sunray appearance

Ans. is 'c' Soap-bubble

49. Which of the following hone tumour present secondaries in lung with pneumothorax: *(AIIMS Sept 96)*

a. Osteosarcoma b. Ewing sarcoma

c. Osteoclastoma d. Chondroblastoma

Ans. is 'a' Osteosarcoma

50. A Pt presents with pneumothorax, Examination shows a swelling over knee. Chest X-ray shows lung nodules, give your most probable diagnosis: *(AIIMS Dec 95)*

a. Osteosarcoma b. Ewing sarcoma

c. Multiple myeloma d. Osteoclastoma

Ans. is 'a' Osteosarcoma

51. Management plan for osteogenic sarcoma of the lower end of femur must include: *(AI 04)*

a. Radiotherapy, amputation, chemotherapy
b. Surgery alone
c. Chemotherapy + Limb Salvage Surgery Chemotherapy
d. Chemotherapy + Radiotherapy

Ans. is 'c' Chemotherapy + Limb Salvage Surgery Chemotherapy

52. A 7-year-old child presents with a lesion in upper tibia. X-ray shows radiolucent area with Codman's triangle and Sunray appearance. Diagnosis is: *(AIIMS May 07, AI 07, NEET/DNB Pattern)*

a. Ewing sarcoma
b. Osteosarcoma
c. Osteoid osteoma
d. Chondrosarcoma

Ans. is 'b' Osteosarcoma

53. Radiological investigation shows sun ray appearance; diagnosis is: *(AIIMS Dec 95)*

a. Osteosarcoma
b. GCT
c. Osteomyelitis
d. Ewing's sarcoma

Ans. is 'a' Osteosarcoma

54. Which of the following malignant tumors is radio resistant:

a. Ewing's sarcoma
b. Retinoblastoma
c. Osteosarcoma
d. Neuroblastoma

Ans. is 'c' Osteosarcoma

55. A 15-year-old boy is injured while playing cricket. X-rays of the leg rule out of a possible fracture. The radiologist reports the boy has an evidence of aggressive bone tumor with both bone destruction and soft tissue mass. The bone biopsy reveals a bone cancer with neural differentiation. Which of the following is the most likely diagnosis? *(AIIMS May 06)*

a. Chondroblastoma
b. Ewing's sarcoma
c. Neuroblastoma
d. Osteosarcoma

Ans. is 'b' Ewing's sarcoma

56. Onion peel appearance in X-ray suggests: *(DPG Feb. 09)*

a. Osteogenic sarcoma b. Ewing's sarcoma

c. Osteoclastoma d. Chondrosarcoma

Ans. is 'b' Ewing's sarcoma

57. Characteristic radiological feature of fibrous dysplasia:

a. Thickened bone matrix *(AIIMS May 10)*

b. Cortical erosion

c. Ground glass appearance

d. Bone enlargement

Ans. is 'c' Ground glass appearance

58. Most common site of adamantinoma of the long bones is: *(AIIMS May 01)*

a. Femur b. Ulna

c. Tibia d. Fibula

Ans. is 'c' Tibia

59. Most common cause of bone malignancy: *(PGI June 08)*

a. Secondaries b. Osteosarcoma

c. Ewing's sarcoma d. Osteoclastoma

Ans. is 'a' Secondaries

60. Expansile lytic osseous metastases are characteristics of primary malignancy of:

a. Kidney b. Bronchus

c. Breast d. Prostate

Ans. is 'a' Kidney

61. Babloo a 10 year old boy presents with # of humerus. X-ray reveals a lytic lesion at the upper end. likely condition is - (AI 01. AIIMS Nov 99)

a. Unicameral bone cyst b. Osteosarcoma

c. Osteoclastoma d. Aneurysmal bone cyst

Ans. is 'a' Unicameral bone cyst

62. Striated vertebra is seen in: *(NEET/DNB Pattern)*

a. TB spine b. Haemangioma

c. Chordoma d. Metastasis

Ans. is 'b' Haemangioma

Chapter 5

Fracture and Fracture Healing

ANATOMY OF BONE

Major Bone mineral is Hydroxyapatite.

In children, a typical long bone has two ends or epiphyses an **intermediate portion diaphysis** connecting part between the two metaphysis. There is a thin plate of growth cartilage one at each end, separating the epiphysis from the metaphysis. This is called the Physeal plate. At maturity, the epiphysis fuses with the metaphysis and the Physeal plate is replaced by bone. The articular ends of the epiphyses are covered with articular cartilage. The rest of the bone is covered with periosteum which provides attachment to tendons, muscles, ligaments etc. The strands of fibrous tissue connecting the bone to the periosteum are called Sharpey's fibers.

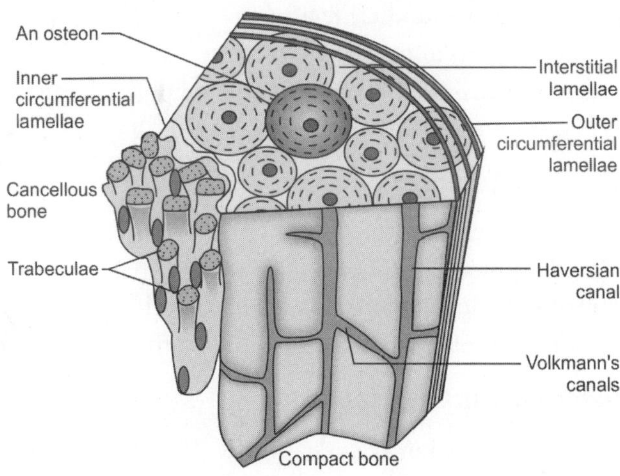

Fig. 5.1: Bone

Microscopically, bone can be classified as either woven or lamellar.

Woven bone or immature bone is characterized by random arrangement of cells and collagen it is associated with periods of rapid bone formation, such as in the **initial stages of fracture healing**.

Lamellar bone or mature bone has an orderly cellular distribution and properly oriented collagen fibres. The **basic structural unit of lamellar bone is the osteon**. It consists of a series of concentric laminations or lamellae surrounding a central canal, the Haversian canal. These canals run longitudinally and connect freely with each other and with Volkmann's canals, which run horizontally from endosteal to periosteal surfaces. The lamellae may be arranged densely to form the cortical bone, or loosely to form the cancellous bone. The shaft of a bone is made up of cortical bone; the ends mainly of cancellous bone. The junction between the two known as cortico - cancellous junction is a common site of fractures.

Growth of a Long Bone

1. Limbs appear at the end of 1st month of intrauterine life.
2. All long bones, with the exception of the clavicle, develop from cartilaginous primordia (enchondral ossification).

This type of ossification commences in the middle of the shaft (primary centre of ossification) before birth usually beginning by the end of 2nd month of intrauterine life.

3. Muscles and joints appear in 3rd month.
4. The secondary ossification centers (the epiphyses) appear at the ends of the bone, mostly around and after birth.

Endochondral Ossification

- When bone formation takes pace in preexisting cartilage.
- The cartilage model formed from mesenchymal tissue acts as a scaffold for ossification but does not itself become bone.
- Long bones, vertebrae, pelvis, and bones of the base of skull.

Intramembranous Ossification

- When bone formation occurs directly in primitive connective tissue by proliferation, hypertrophy and transformation of cells into osteoblasts .

- Progressive bone formation results in the fusion of adjacent bony areas within the membrane to form spongy bone
- Skull vault, maxilla, majority of mandible and clavicle.

The bone grows in length by a continuous growth at the Epiphyseal plate. The increase in the girth of the bone is by subperiosteal new bone deposition. The secondary centers of ossification, not contributing to the length of a bone, are termed the apophysis (e.g., apophysis. of the greater trochanter). At the end of the growth period, the epiphysis fuses with the metaphysis and the growth stops. The time and sequence of appearance and fusion of epiphysis has great clinical relevance in deciding the true age (bone age) of a person, and in differentiating an Epiphyseal plate from a fracture.

Milking position to remember age of ossification or skeletal maturity – **Joints that face towards sky or god like shoulder/wrist/ knee usually ossify around 18 and joints that face towards ground like elbow/hip and ankle fuse around 16.**

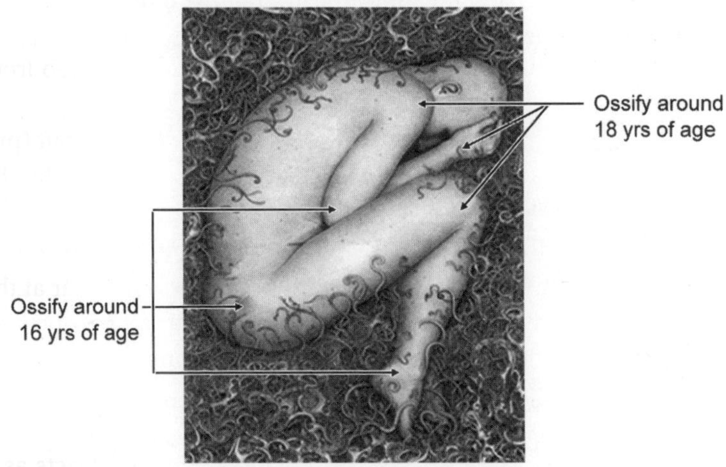

Fig. 5.2: Milking position

Cells of Bone

Oteoblast

- Mononuclear cells are derived from marrow stromal cells by differentiation of preosteoblasts. The single nucleus is eccentrically placed and the abundant rough endoplasmic reticulum (RER) is characteristic of a cell engaged in protein synthesis. They are rich in alkaline phosphatase.

- It is responsible for the synthesis of major protein of bone including type I collagen and non collagen proteins such as — osteocalcin. (bone Gla protein) and osteonectin. **It plays a central role in osteoclastic function (i.e. involved in initiation and control of osteoclastic activity)** Osteoblasts have specific surface recceptors for 1, 25- Dihydroxy vitamin D3 and Parathyroid hormone.

Osteocytes

- By the end of bone remodelling cycle, the osteoblast either remains on newly formed surface as quiescent lining cell or become enveloped in the matrix as resting osteocytes. So **these are spent osteoblasts.**
- Their function is obscure : they may under the influence of PTH, participate in bone resorption (osteocytic osteolysis) and calcium ion transport.

Osteoclast

- It is multinucleated giant cell
- It is the principal mediator of bone resorption and is **formed by fusion of mononuclear cells.**
- The characteristic feature is the area of in folded plasma membrane ruffled border which is the site of bone resorption.
- In order to create this enclosed space, the osteoclast attaches to the bone through special attachment proteins called integrins.
- It contain characteristic enzymes Tartrate resistant acid phosphatase (TRAP) and carbonic anhydrase
- With resorption of organic matrix, the osteoclasts are left in shallow excavations- Howship's lacunae in cancellous bone and cutting cones in cortical bones. By identifying these excavations one can distinguish 'resorption surface' from the smooth 'formation surface' or 'resting surface.

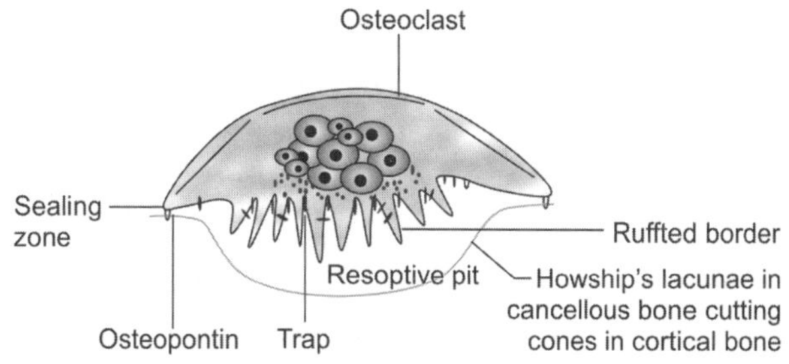

Fig. 5.3: Osteoclast

Note: Osteoid mineralization is assessed by Tetracycline labelling.

FRACTURE: DIAGNOSIS AND PATTERN

Radiological Feature

Partial or complete loss of continuity of cortex .

Clinical Features

Tenderness is the commonest sign of fracture.

Abnormal mobility and loss of transmitted movements is surest sign of fracture. If these two are not mentioned than crepitus should be marked as the answer.

* Crepitus occurs because of rubbing of both fracture ends together and gives sense of friction between fractured ends, it should not be elicited as it may cause neurogenic shock or may cause comminution at fracture ends due to rubbing of bone ends. Crepitus may also be positive in bursitis or subcutaneous emphysema. Thus crepitus is not a reliable sign of fracture.

Fracture

Pathological :	**The broken bone has an underlying disease most common cause in India is nutritional disorder.**
Comminuted :	Fracture in multiple pieces and intermediate fragment has only one cortex
Segmental :	Fracture at two levels in the same bone with intermediate segment having two cortices.
Avulsion :	Bone piece pulled-off by attached muscle or ligament
Burst :	Vertebral body fracture where fragments burst out in different directions - Compression injury

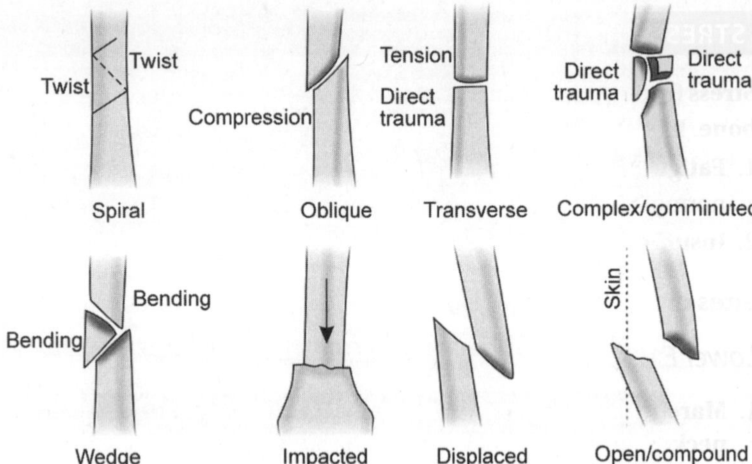

Fig. 5.4: Fracture pattern and mode of injury

- Fractures can be Classified on basis of **Pattern of injury**
- **Transverse fractures (fracture forms an angle of less than 30 degrees with horizontal)** - Tension/direct trauma
- **Oblique fractures (fracture forms an angle of more than 30 degrees with horizontal)** - Compression injury
- **Spiral fractures** - Twisting injury and it has maximum chances of union
- **Bending - Butterfly (Comminuted) fracture**
- **Direct - Comminuted fracture**
- **Direct trauma - Transverse > Comminuted fracture**

FRACTURE CLASSIFICATION ON THE BASIS OF RELATIONSHIP WITH EXTERNAL ENVIRONMENT

Closed Fracture

A fracture hematoma not comminucating with external environment i.e. overlying skin and soft tissue are intact.

Open Fracture

A fracture hematoma communicating with external environment i.e. over lying skin (and soft tissue) is breached.

Gustilo and Anderson Classification is used for open fracture

STRESS/FATIGUE FRACTURE

Stress fracture is due to imbalance between load and resistance of bone. It is of 2 types:

1. **Fatigue Fracture:** Caused by application of abnormal stress on normal bone.
2. **Insufficiency Fracture:** Caused by normal activity on weak bone.

Sites of Stress Fractures

Lower Extremity

1. **March fracture is a** stress fatigue fracture of second metatarsal **neck. > 3rd metatarsal neck.**

   The most common site is metatarsal neck followed by tibia (proximal third in children, middle third in athlete and lower third in elderly).
2. Femoral neck
3. Rarely fibula lower end **(runners fracture)**

Upper Extremity

- **Olecranon** is most common site of upper limb stress fractures.

Pelvis and Spine

- **Pars inter articularis of 5th lumbar vertebral (causing spondylolysis) is commonest in spine**.

Clinical Presentation

- Load related pain often bilateral
- The hallmark physical finding is tenderness with palpation and stress.

Investigation

- MRI provide excellent sensitivity and superior specificity compared to bone scan in differentiating from infections or tumors.
- Bone scan is preferable for bilateral cases due to feasibility, also bilateral cases go in favour of stress fracture as compared to Infection or tumor and also can scan the whole body.

- Treatment is symptomatic with cast and cessation of activity
- **Markers of Bone formation**
  Serum bone specific alkaline phosphatase
  Serum osteocalcin (very important marker)
- **Markers of Bone Resorption**
  Urine hydroxyproline
  Serum tartrate-resistant acid phosphatase (TRAP)

Common Sites of Nonunion

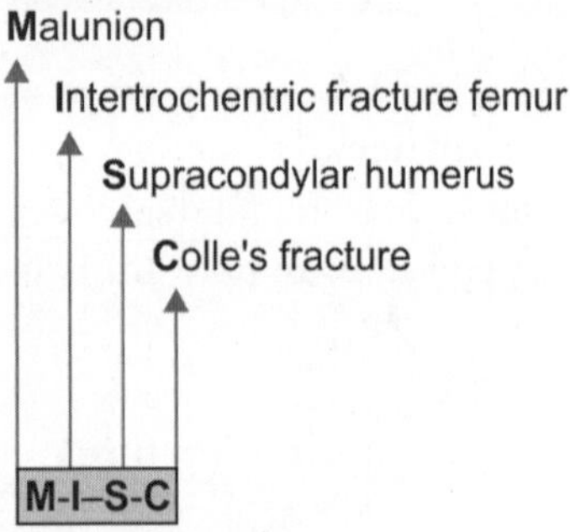

Common sites of Malunion

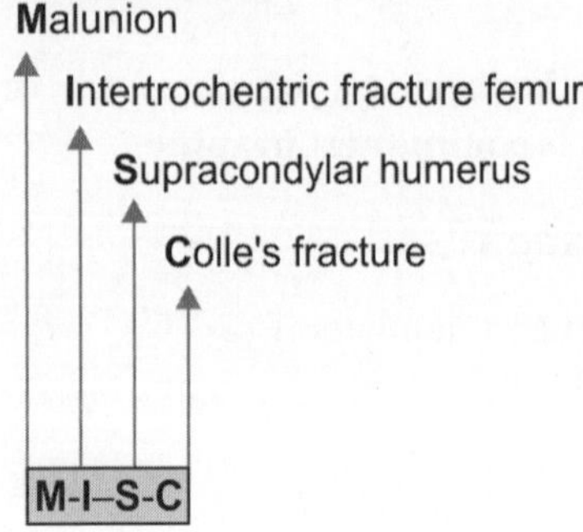

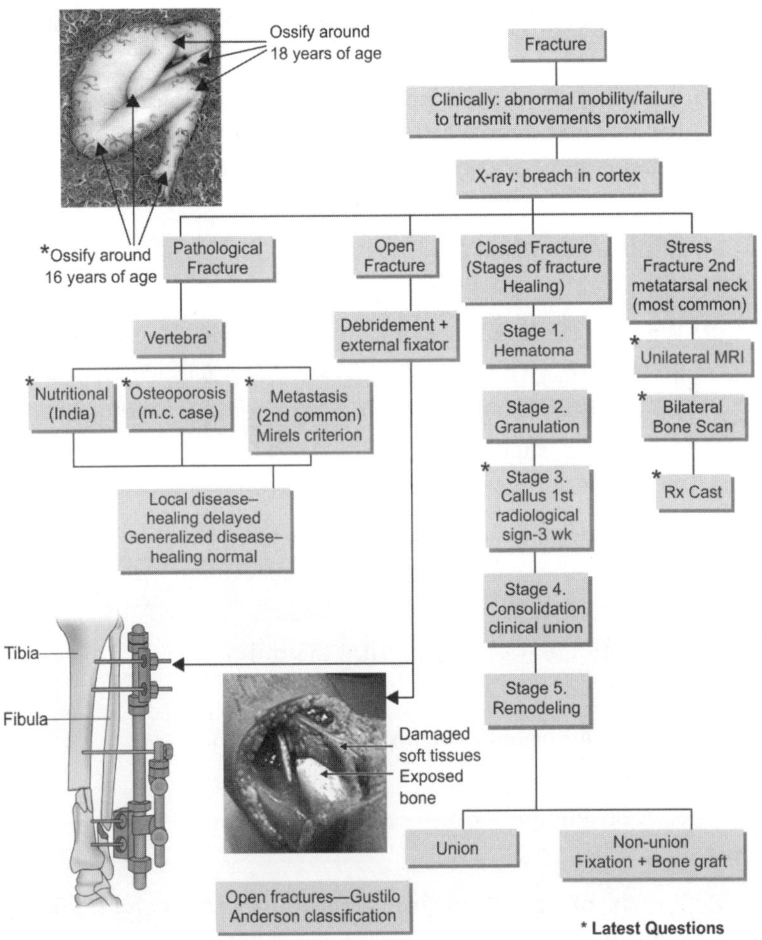

* **Latest Questions**

QUESTIONS

1. A male patient presents after trauma with popliteal vessel injury and fracture of 0.5 cm × 0.5 cm. What is the Anderson Gustilo classification? *(Recent Pattern Question 2017)*

a. 1 b. 2

c. 3A d. 3C

Ans. is 'd' 3C

2. What is the treatment of Anderson Gustilo classification grade 3B? *(Recent Pattern Question 2017)*

a. Intramedullary nailing b. Intramedullary wiring

c. Close reduction d. Debridement

Ans. is 'd' Debridement

3. Connection of Haversian canal are by *(Recent Pattern Question 2017)*

a. Canaliculi b. Volkmann canal

c. Osteon d. Central canal

Ans. is 'b' Volkmann canal

4. Stress fracture occurs most commonly in:

a. Metatarsals b. Metacarpals

c. Calcaneum d. Talus

Ans. is 'a' Metatarsals

5. Which of the following fracture most likely leads to malunion:

a. Clavicle fracture b. Femur neck fracture

c. Scaphoid fracture d. Ulna fracture

Ans. is 'a' Clavicle fracture

6. Correct meaning of Poncet disease:

a. TB with Rheumatoid arthritis

b. TB of short bones

c. TB with polyarthritis

d. TB of shoulder

Ans. is 'c' TB with polyarthritis

7. Major mineral of the bone is: *(AIIMS May 10)*

a. Calcite
b. Hydroxyapatite
c. Calcium oxide
d. Calcium carbonate

Ans. is 'b' Hydroxyapatite

8. Which of the changes occur in bone growth: *(AIIMS Dec 97)*

a. Increased acid phosphatase
b. Increased urinary calcium
c. Increased bone nucleotidase
d. Increased osteocalcin

Ans. is 'd' Increased osteocalcin

9. Indicators of bone formation includes all of following except: *(AI 07, 11)*

a. Osteocalcin
b. Alkaline phosphatase
c. Hydroxyproline
d. Type 1 procollagen

Ans. is 'c' Hydroxyproline

10. Rate of newly synthesized osteoid mineralization can be best estimated by: *(AI 09)*

a. Tetracycline labeling
b. Alizarin red stain
c. Calcein stain
d. Von Kossa stain

Ans. is 'a' Tetracycline labeling

11. Stress fracture not Involved is: *(PGI 00)*

a. Metatarsals
b. Metacarpals
c. Tibia
d. Calcaneum

Ans. is 'b' Metacarpals

12. Commonest site of March fracture is: *(PGI June 2K)*

a. Involves 2 & 3" metatarsals
b. Avulsion # of 5th metatarsals
c. Calcaneus involved
d. Olecranon involved

Ans. is 'a' Involves 2 & 3" metatarsals

13. What is March fracture? *(PGI 99. NEET/DNB Pattern)*

a. Fracture of 2nd metatarsal
b. Fracture of 4th metatarsal
c. Fracture of cuboids
d. Fracture of tibia

Ans. is 'a' Fracture of 2nd metatarsal

14. Non-union is a complication of: *(AIIMS June 98 NEET/DNB Pattern)*

a. Scaphoid fracture
b. Colle's fracture
c. Inter-trochanteric fracture of hip
d. Supracondylar fracture of humerus

Ans. is 'a' Scaphoid fracture

15. The following fractures are known for Non-union except: *(DNB 90, UP 02)*

a. Fracture of lower half of tibia
b. Fracture of neck of femur
c. Fracture of scaphoid
d. Fracture of patella
e. Supracondylar fracture of humerus

Ans. is 'e' Supracondylar fracture of humerus (This fracture is known as for malunion)

Chapter 6

Advanced Trauma Life Support

Any trauma patient should be managed in following sequent of events (ABCDEF):

A. Airway management with cervical spine stabilization (Cervical spine stabilization before Airway)

B. Breathing (ventilation)

C. Circulation

D. Disability (neurological status) assessment

E. Exposure and environmental control

F. Fracture splintage

QUESTION

1. **On accident there is damage of cervical spine, first line of management is:** *(AIIMS Nov 99, PGI 94, NEET/DNB Pattern)*
   a. X-ray
   b. Turn head to side
   c. Maintain airway
   d. Stabilise the cervical spine

Ans. is 'd' Stabilise the cervical spine

Chapter 7

Upper Limb Traumatology

SHOULDER ANATOMY

Normal function of the shoulder is a balance between mobility and stability. **The bony anatomy contributes little to stability and has been compared with a golf ball on a tee.** The bony anatomy of the shoulder joint does not provide inherent stability. The glenoid fossa is a flattened, dishlike structure. **Only one fourth of the large humeral head articulates with the glenoid at any given time.** The glenoid is encircled by the labrum, a dense fibrocartilaginous tissue, which increases the depth of the socket by 50% around the humeral head and increases stability.

Integral to the glenoid labrum is the insertion of the tendon of the long head of the biceps, which inserts on the superior aspect of the joint and blends to become indistinguishable from the posterior glenoid labrum.

Four rotator cuff muscles are—supraspinatus, infraspinatus, subscapularis and teres minor.

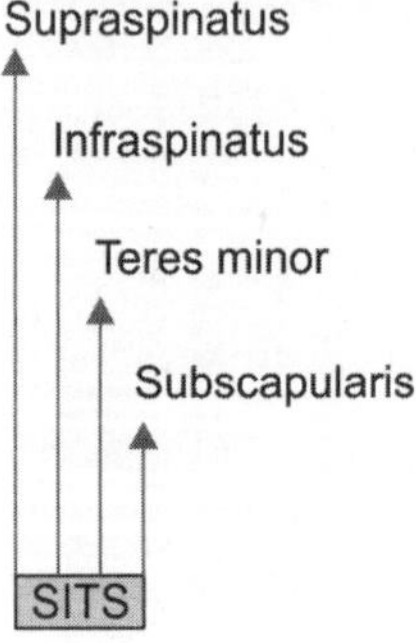

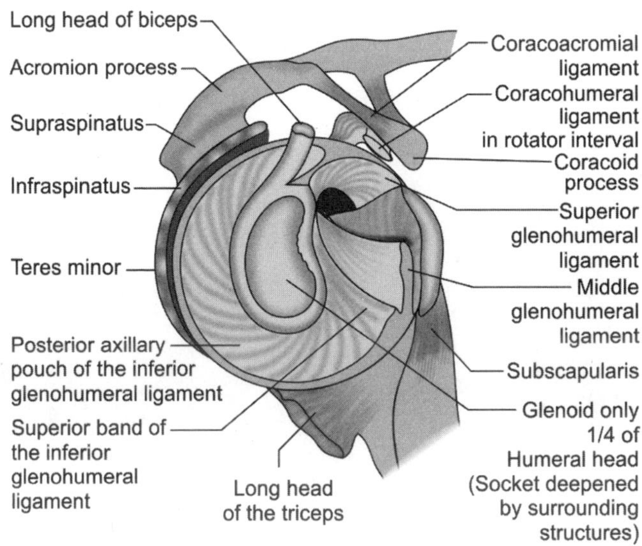

Fig. 7.1: Anatomy of shoulder

The tendon of rotator cuff muscles blend with the joint capsule and form a musculo tendinous collar that surrounds the posterior, superior, and anterior aspect of gleno- humeral joint. **The inferior part of shoulder joint capsule is the weakest area.**

The tendon of the long head of biceps brachii muscle passes superiorly through the joint and restricts upward movement of humeral head on glenoid cavity.

Rotator interval is interval between leading edge of supraspinatus and superior edge of subscapularis. Coracohumeral ligament passes within rotator interval.

LIFT OFF TEST (GERBER'S TEST)

Lift off test is done to assess the strength of subscapularis muscle and detect a rupture of the subscapularis tendon. Subscapularis functions primarily as an internal rotator of the shoulder. The test is performed with the arm extended and internally rotated such that the dorsum of the hand rests against the lower back. Subscapularis is maximally active in this position. Patient is then instructed to lift his/her hand off the back (Lift-off) (Attempting further internal rotation). If the patient is able to lift the dorsum of the hand off the back the subscapularis tendon is intact and the test is considered negative.

If the patient is not able to lift the dorsum of the hand off the back the subscapularis tendon is torn and the test is considered positive.

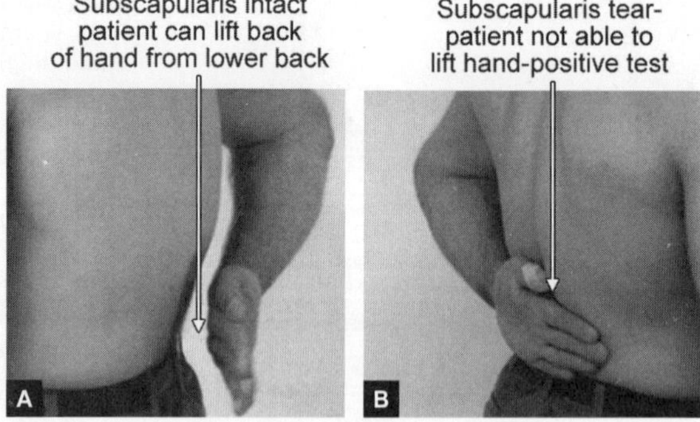

Figs. 7.2A and B: Lift off test

Lesions associated with recurrent dislocation.

1. Bankart's Lesion:

In 1938, Bankart published his classic paper in which he recognized two types of acute dislocations. In the first type, the humeral head is forced through the capsule where it is the weakest, generally anteriorly and inferiorly in the interval between the lower border of the subscapularis and the long head of the triceps muscle. In the second type, the humeral head is forced anteriorly out of the glenoid cavity and tears not only the fibrocartilaginous labrum from almost the entire anterior half of the rim of the glenoid cavity, but also the capsule and periosteum from the anterior surface of the neck of the scapula. This traumatic detachment of the glenoid labrum has been called the Bankart lesion. Most authors agree that the Bankart lesion is the most commonly observed pathological lesion in recurrent subluxation or dislocation of the shoulder.

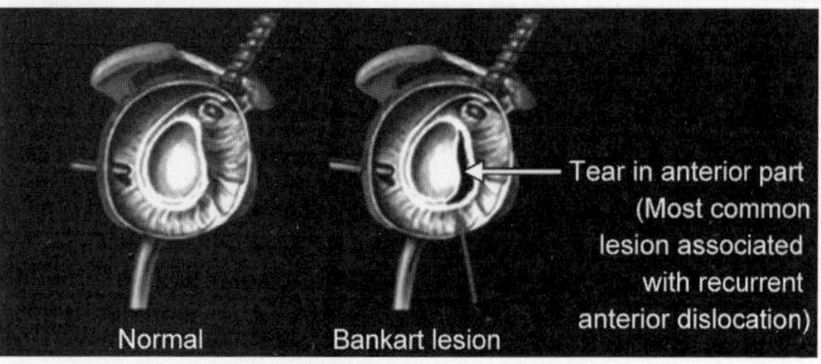

Fig. 7.3: Bankart lesion

2. Hill-Sach's lesion:

A humeral head impaction fracture can be produced as the shoulder is dislocated anteriorly, and the humeral head is impacted against the rim of the glenoid at the time of dislocation. This Hill-Sachs lesion is a defect in the posterolateral aspect of the humeral head. If these lesions involve more than 20% of the glenoid, they can result in recurrent instability despite having an excellent soft-tissue repair. They are also called as impression fractures.

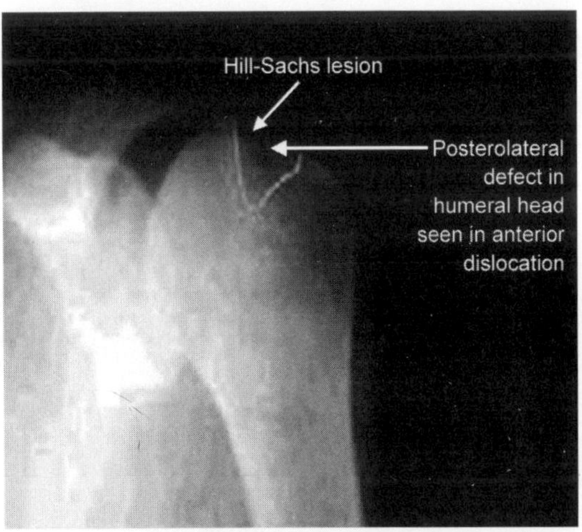

Fig. 7.4: Hill-Sachs lesion

Note: Reverse Hill. Sachs lesion is associated with posterior dislocation of shoulder

MODE OF INJURY CAUSING SHOULDER DISLOCATION

Recurrent anterior dislocation: Abduction and External rotation force

Posterior dislocation: Indirect force producing marked internal rotation and adduction

Inferior dislocation: Severe hyperabduction force

1. Salute position

Anterior Dislocation of Shoulder-Most common type of shoulder dislocation

Mechanism of Injury: Abduction and External Rotation Force

Types: Subcoracoid > Preglenoid > Subclavicular

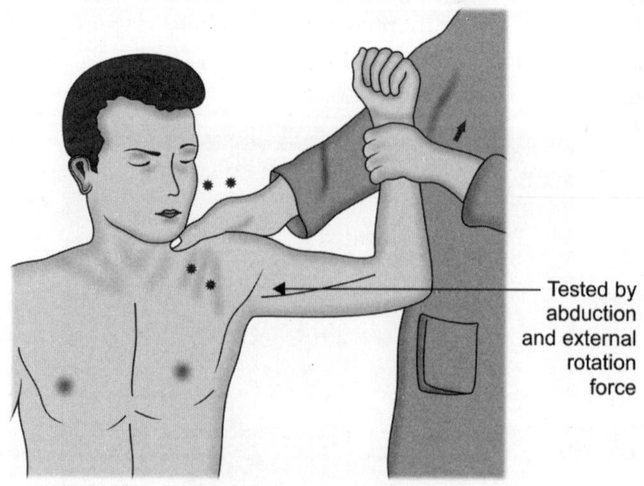

Fig. 7.5: Anterior instability

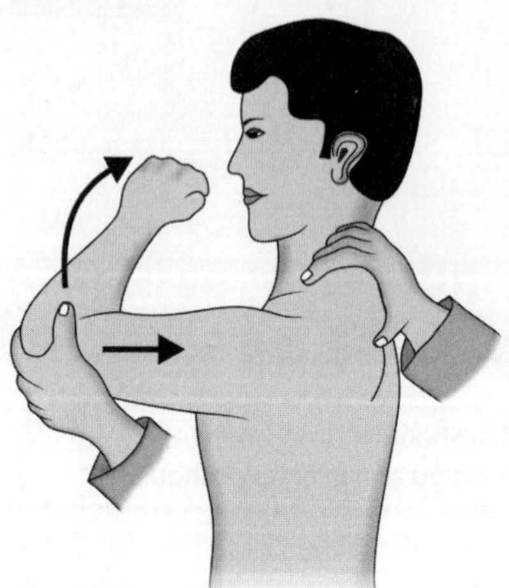

Fig. 7.6: Jerk test (Posterior instability)

Clinical Features

- Patient keeps his arm slightly abducted. (Based on Location of Humeral head)
- Normal round contour of shoulder is lost and it becomes flat.

1. *Bryant's test:* Anterior axillary fold is at lower level.
2. *Dugas test:* It is not possible for the patient to bring the elbow close to the body and touch the tip of opposite shoulder.
3. *Callaway's test:* Vertical circumference of axilla is increased as compared to the normal side.
4. *Hamilton ruler test:* Because of flattening of shoulder, it is possible to place a ruler on the lateral side of arm and it touches acromian and lateral condyle of humerus simultaneously (in normal it would not due to shoulder contour).

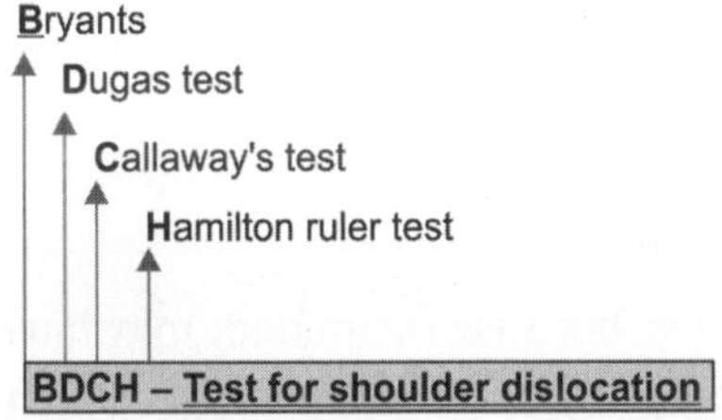

- A -P X-ray show overlapping shadow of humeral head and glenoid fossa; and lateral view show humeral head Out of line with the socket.

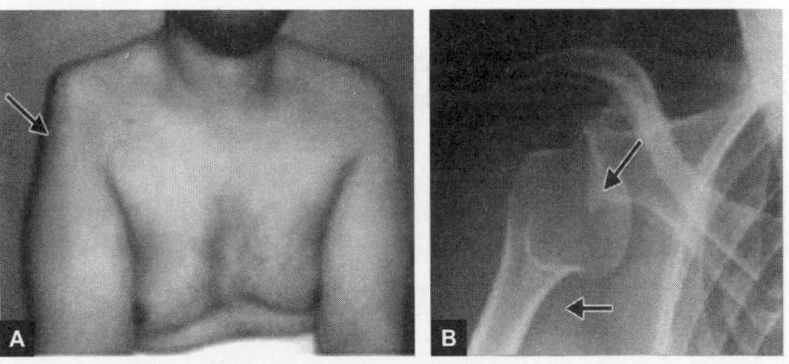

Figs. 7.7A and B: Shoulder dislocation (A) Lost contour of shoulder; (B) Abducted arm in anterior shoulder dislocation

Management

- Commonly used reduction techniques are Stimson's gravity method, Hippocratic method and Kocher's method.

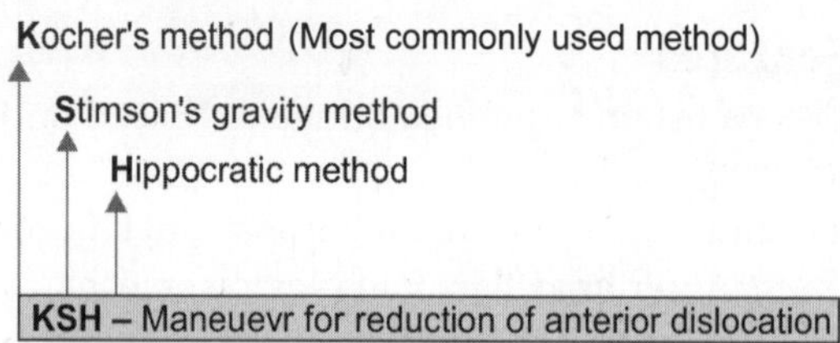

- **Kochers method** is done by traction in slight abduction and external rotation to increase deformity followed by adduction and internal rotation. Post reduction there is positioning of the limb in adduction and internal rotation called as chest arm bandage × 3 weeks.

"Most common early complication of anterior dislocation of shoulder is nerve injury"

Most commonly injured nerve in anterior dislocation of shoulder is circumflex branch of axillary nerve. The injury to nerve is usually neuropraxia

Inferior dislocation also axillary nerve involvement is commonest.

2. Posterior Dislocation

Difficult to diagnose because the patient may have normal contour of shoulder. Holds injured **shoulder in internal rotation** and examiner cannot externally rotate it.

3. Inferior Dislocation (Luxatio erecta / Subglenoid)

Locked in full abduction, fixed by the side of head.

INJURIES AROUND ELBOW

Elbow Anatomy

- Capitellum is the first ossification centre about the elbow to appear. It appears around 2 years of age.
- The mnemonic "CRITOE" is helpful in remembering the progression of the radiographic appearance of ossification centre about the elbow in children:
  - **C** : Capitellum – 2 years
  - **R** : Radius head – 4 years
  - **I** : Internal (medial) epicondyle – 6 years
  - **T** : Trochlea – 8 years
  - **O** : Olecranon – 10 years
  - **E** : External (Lateral) epicondyle – 12 years

Carrying angle: Angle between long axis of arm and forearm. angle is more in females because of lower level of trochlea in female. Normal value is 5-15°. Cubitus Varus is reduced carrying angle and cubitus valgus is increased carrying angle. Varus - distal part towards midline and valgus is distal part away from midline.

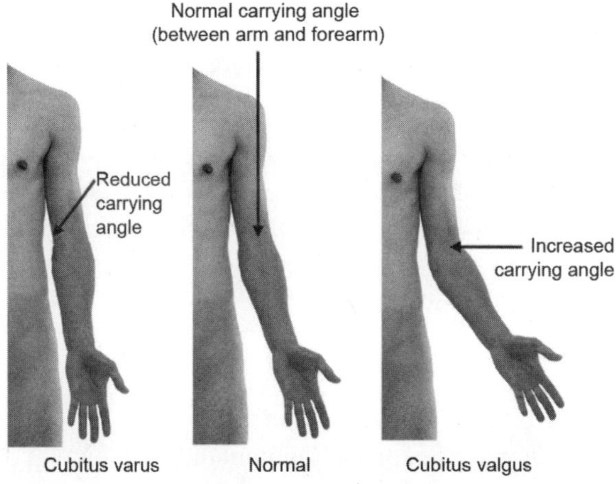

Fig. 7.8: Carrying angle

Note : Malunion around elbow causes Varus=cubitus (elbow) varus

Nonunion around elbow causes valgus =cubitus valgus

Supracondylar fracture humerus -causes malunion hence cubitus varus

Lateral condyle fracture humerus is known for nonunion and it involves growth plate hence it causes cubitus valgus that can be progressive.

Three Point Bony Landmarks In Elbow

- The tips of medial and lateral epicondyles and the olecranon.
- Form Isosceles triangle – **In Elbow flexion of 90 degree.**
- **Lie transversely in straight line – Elbow Extension.**
- ***Three point bony relationship is not disturbed in fracture supracondylar humerus as the fracture occurs above the level of these bony landmarks.***

A. With disturbed (increased) intercondylar distance

Fracture lateral epicondyle and condyle

Fracture medial epicondyle and condyle

Fracture intercondylar humerus.

B. With maintained intercondylar distance

Elbow dislocation (classical example)

Fracture olecranon (i.e. upper end ulna)

- Weak posterior capsule may disrupt three point bony relation by promoting subluxation or dislocations of elbow.

Radial head, lateral epicondyle and tip of olecranon form a triangle over the posterolateral aspect of elbow joint. This space is occupied by anconeus muscle and so known as **anconeus triangle**.

FRACTURE SUPRACONDYLAR HUMERUS

Supracondylar humeral fractures in children are most common elbow injuries, especially in children aged 5-8 years. They account for 50 — 70% of all elbow fractures.

Mechanism

- Most common type of supracondylar fracture-Extension type (~98% of all supracondylar fracture).
- Most common type of distal fragment displacement in extension type fracture supracondylar humerus

"Posteromedial displacement with internal rotation"

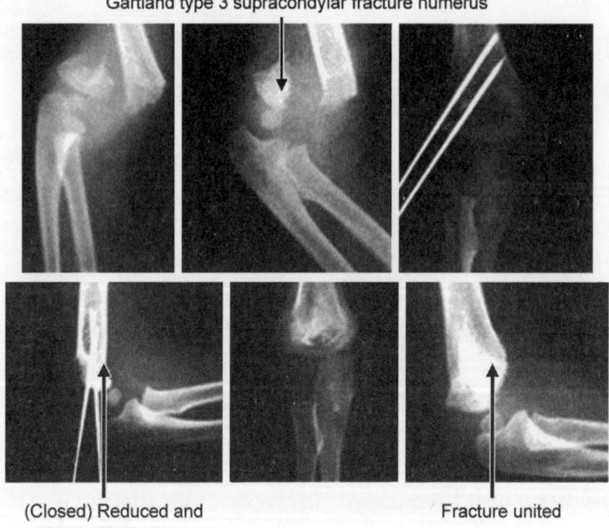

Fig. 7.9: Displaced supracondylar fracture humerus and its treatment with K-wires.

- Most common type of displacement in flexion type (2%) fracture supracondylar humerus Anterior displacement

Gartland Classification is Used for Supracondylar fractures

- **Treatment is closed reduction and cast if it fails or if fracture is displaced than closed reduction and K-wire fixation.**
- **Admission to Hospital is Essential following Reduction:**

Potential problem with close reduction and cast management of fracture supra condylar humerus is increased swelling and potential development of compartment syndrome, hence they require observation.

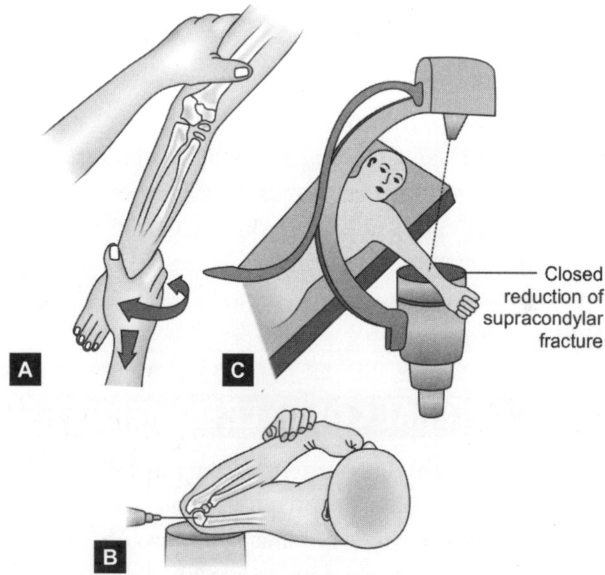

Figs. 7.10A to C: Closed reduction and fixation

Complications of Fracture Supracondylar Humerus

1. Malunion Most Common Complication

Posteromedially displaced fracture tend to develop Cubitus varus (gun stock deformity).

- Cubitus varus deformity in Fracture supracondylar humerus is managed by French/modified French osteotomy (lateral close wedge osteotomy).

2. Vascular (brachial artery) injury
3. Nerve injury (anterior interosseous n.> median n. > radial n > ulnar. n)

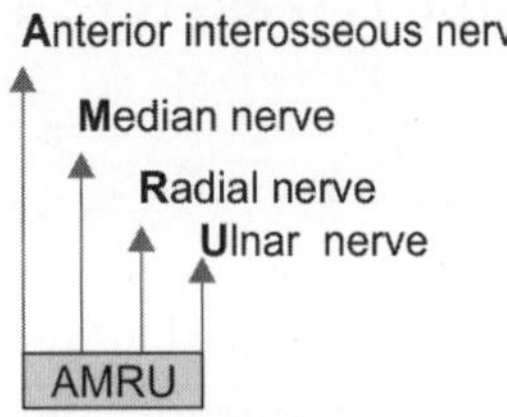

4. Volkman's ischemia and compartment syndrome
5. Elbow stiffness
6. Myositis ossificans
7. Avascular necrosis of trochlea. (rare)
8. Tardy ulnar nerve palsy

Fracture supracondylar humerus is
- Most common fracture associated with vascular injury.
- Most common fracture to involve brachial artery. (10% cases)
- Most common cause of Volkmann's ischemia and compartment syndrome in children.
- Most common cause of Volkmann's ischemic contracture
- Non-union is unknown

FRACTURE LATERAL CONDYLE HUMERUS

- This is a transphyseal intra-articular injury usually involving immature skeleton of children and adolescent.
- The lateral condylar (or capitellar) epiphysis begins to ossify during the first year of life and fuses with shaft at 12-16 years. Between these ages it may be sheared off or avulsed by forceful traction. The maximum chances of injury is between 5—15 years.

  They are the **most common distal humeral epiphyseal fracture.**

  Mechanism of Fracture Lateral Condyle Humerus Fall on outstretched arm with Varus stress (mostly) that "Pulls off" (avulses) lateral condyle or Valgus force (rarely) in which radial head directly pushes off the lateral condyle.

  Milch described two basic types of lateral condylar fractures.

Results are unsatisfactory after closed treatment so open reduction and internal fixation with K-wires/screws is necessary – hence the term *fracture of necessity.*

> **Fractures of necessity (requiring surgery)**
> - *Lateral condyle fracture humerus*
> - *Displaced fracture olecranon and patella*
> - *Fracture neck femur*
> - *Galeazzi fracture dislocation*
> - *Monteggia fracture in adults*
> - *Articular fractures*

1. **Nonunion is most frequent problematic complication.**
- **The most common sequela of nonunion with displacement is the development of progressive cubitus valgus deformity.**
- Treatment of cubitus valgus –Milch Osteotomy.
2. Tardy ulnar nerve palsy is a late complication of progressive cubitus valgus>cubitus varus deformity occuring in lateral condylar fractures.

Tardy Ulnar Nerve Palsy

Tardy ulnar nerve palsy as a late complication of fracture lateral condyle physis is well known, after the development of cubitus valgus.

The symptoms are usually gradual in onset and may appear years after injury. Motor loss occur first, with sensory changes developing later.

Anterior transposition of ulnar nerve is most commonly used procedure.

COMPARTMENT SYNDROME-TIGHT CAST THINK OF COMPARTMENT SYNDROME

In acute compartment syndromes increased pressure in a close fascial space causes loss of microcirculation.

Most commonly compartment syndrome involves deep posterior compartment of leg>deep flexor compartment of forearm (commonest in children).

It is most commonly seen following fractures of supracondylar humerus and tibia.

Most common cause is fractures and dislocations: Other Causes of compartment syndrome

1. **Crush injury/Burn**/Infection/**Surgical procedure/Tight circumferential dressing**
2. **Exercise**-Exercise may increase intra compartmental pressure and muscle edema, so it is avoided in cases of acute compartmental syndrome.

Clinical Features

The diagnosis of compartment syndrome is based on dramatically increasing pain (out of proportion to injury) after fracture/ any injury (1st symptom).

Pain and resistance on passive stretch (Distal most joint of extremity) (1st sign)

In compartment syndrome the order of compression of vascular structures with increase of intra compartmental pressure is: capillary compression, venous compression, arterial compression. Pulselessness is a late feature and it is not a reliable indicator of compartment syndrome. The presence of pulse does not exclude the diagnosis.

Pressures in the deep volar compartment are significantly elevated compared with pressures in other compartments. **Deep flexor muscles are involved particularly flexor digitorum profundus>Flexor Pollicis Longus.**

Treatment

- **The limb should be kept at the level of heart rather than elevated.**
- **Removed of all circumferential dressing reduce pressure upto 85%**
- Fasciotomy is recommended in the presence of clinical signs of compartment syndrome, such as undue pain and a palpable firmness in the forearm. The morbidity caused by fasciotomy is minimal, whereas that caused by an untreated compartment syndrome is much greater. The general indications for fasciotomy are Impending tissue ischemia or it may be considered when the tissue pressure reaches 30 mm Hg or the difference between diastolic blood pressure and compartment pressure is less than 30 mm of Hg. (normal compartment pressure is 8-10 mm of Hg and pressure at calf during walking is 200 – 300 mm of Hg).

A higher pressure is a strong indication that fasciotomy should be recommended. In a hypotensive patient, the acceptable pressure is lower. Mubarak recommended that fasciotomy be performed in (1) normotensive patients with positive clinical findings, compartment pressures of greater than 30 mm Hg, and when the duration of the increased pressure is unknown or thought to be longer than 8 hours; (2) uncooperative or unconscious patients with a compartment pressure greater than 30 mm Hg; (3) patients with low blood pressure and a compartment pressure greater than 20 mm Hg (4) clinical signs such as demonstrable motor or sensory loss, and (5) interrupted arterial circulation to the extremity for more than 4 hours.

Note: Pallor, Paraesthesias and pulselessness are late signs of compartment syndrome.

Volkmann's Ischaemic Contracture (VIC)

Volkmann's Ischaemic Contracture (VIC): Most commonly in upper limbs (After supracondylar fracture)

If a compartment syndrome is untreated or inadequately treated, compartment pressures continue to increase until irreversible tissue ischemia occurs. In Volkmann ischemic contracture earliest changes usually involve the flexor digitorum profundus muscles in the middle third of the forearm followed by flexor pollicis longus. The typical clinical picture of established Volkmann contracture includes elbow flexion, forearm pronation, wrist flexion, thumb adduction, metacarpophalangeal joint extension, and finger flexion.

The earliest nerve involved is Anterior interossei > median > ulnar

During the early stages of a mild contracture, dynamic splinting (Turn Buckle splint) to prevent wrist contracture, functional training, and active use of the muscles may be helpful. After 3 months, the involved muscle-tendon units can be released and lengthened.

Muscle sliding operation of Flexors for Established Volkmann Contracture

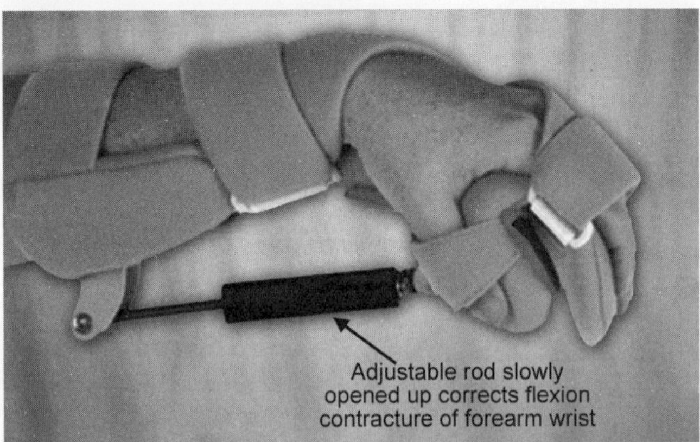

Fig. 7.11: Turn buckle splint - VIC

MYOSITIS OSSIFICANS / HETEROTROPIC OSSIFICATION-HISTORY OF MASSAGE THINK OF IT

It is **hetrotropic calcification and ossification in muscle** tissue. The name is **misnomer as there is no myositis** (inflammation of muscle) and rarely ossification in the muscle (because the mineral phase differs from that in bone and no true bone matrix is formed). Myositis is usually seen in 2nd to 3rd decade of life.

Causes

- **Injury (trauma)** is an important factor when associated with **massage.** Myositis Ossificans is seen in Elbow (MC) followed by hip joint.
- In elbow Myositis is seen more commonly anteriorly than posteriorly
- **Massage to the elbow and vigorous passive stretching to restore movements is aggravating factor.** It occurs in muscles which are vulnerable to heavy loads, such as **brachialis (commonest), biceps.** Surgical trauma specially total hip replacement, is precipitating factor.

X-ray evidence by 3-6 wks of development

There is peripheral ossification and central lucency of the mass (opposite in osteosarcoma).

The mass is usually separated from underlying bone by at least a thin line and lesion are usually located in the diaphysis. if the lesion is in continuity with the bone it is not myositis ossificans and the possibility of tumor or infection arises.

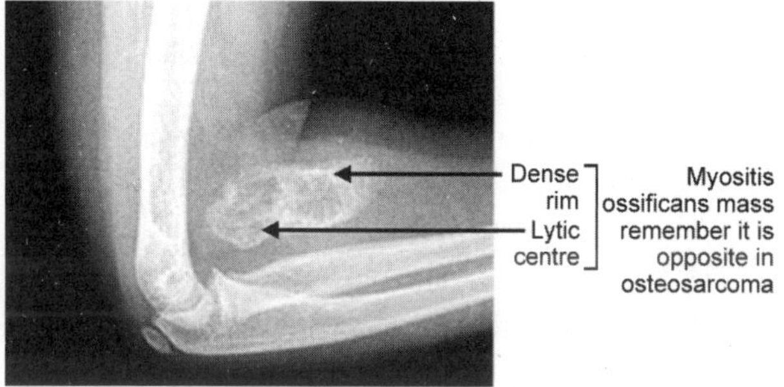

Fig. 7.12: X-ray: elbow- myositis ossificans

Treatment of Myositis Ossificans

In acute phase the treatment consist of limiting motion × **3 weeks. (Immobilization)**

Followed by only active exercises upto 1 year

Surgical excision > 1 year

PULLED ELBOW/ NURSE MAID'S ELBOW

It is subluxation of radial head or more accurately subluxation of the annular (orbicular) ligament which slips up over the head of radius into the radiocapitellar joint.

Mechanism of Injury

Traction to elbow.

Clinical Features

- Maximum incidence in 1-4 years age group.
- The child holds the elbow in slight flexion with the forearm pronated.

X-rays are normal.

Treatment

- Reduced by flexing the elbow to 90 degrees and rapidly and firmly rotating the forearm into full supination **on outdoor basis without anaesthesia** Immobilization is not necessary.

- Supination is a gravity assisted movement and pulled elbow may be reduced spontaneously by gravity, but this may take time.

Colle's Fracture

Colle's fracture is fracture of lower end of radius at its corticocancellous junction mostly occurring in postmenopausal osteoporotic elderly women; as a result of fall on outstretched hand, with wrist in extension . It is one of the most common fracture in elderly.

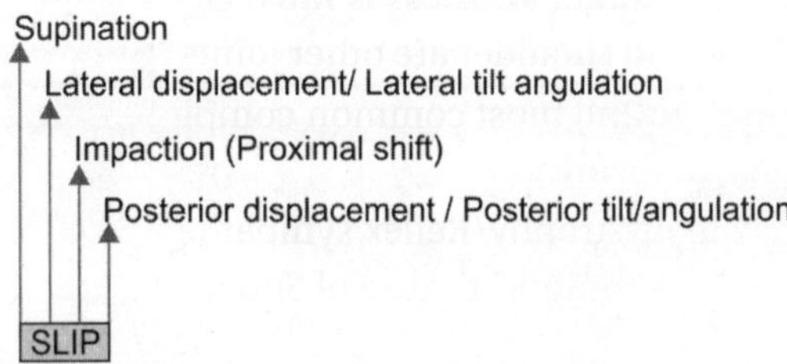

Most Colles fractures can be successfully treated nonoperatively and cast is applied on opposite forces to displacement- That's why position of immobilization in Colle's fracture is

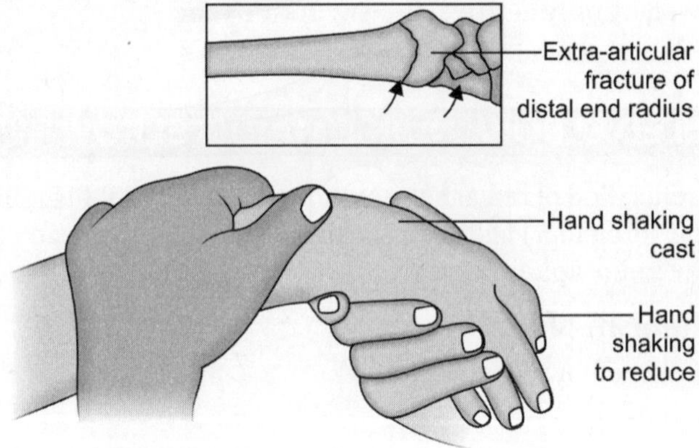

Fig. 7.13: Reduction of colles fracture

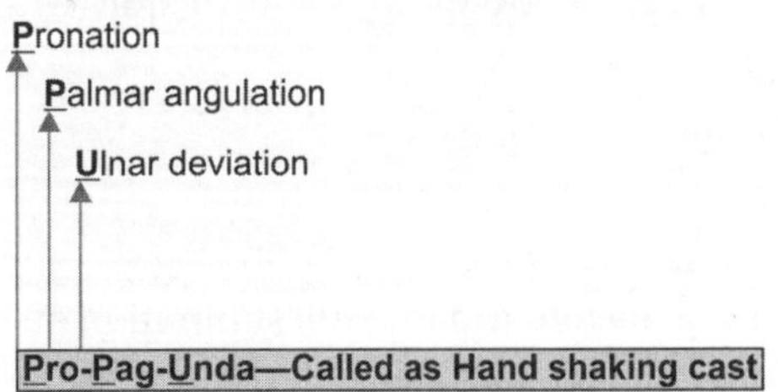

In younger patients, near-normal function and clinical and radiographic appearance are expected. If maintenance of reduction of Colles or Smith fractures requires prolonged immobilization in extreme positions, or reduction is lost early in treatment, closed reduction followed by percutaneous k wire fixation is done.

Complications of Colle's Fracture

- Joint Stiffness: **Finger stiffness is most common complication.** Wrist, elbow, and shoulder are other joints to become stiff.
- Malunion is the 2nd most common complication and it leads to **dinner fork deformity**
- Sudeck's osteodystrophy/Reflex sympathetic dystrophy. Colle's fracture is the commonest cause of Sudeck's dystrophy in upper limb.
- Rupture of extensor pollicis longus tendon.

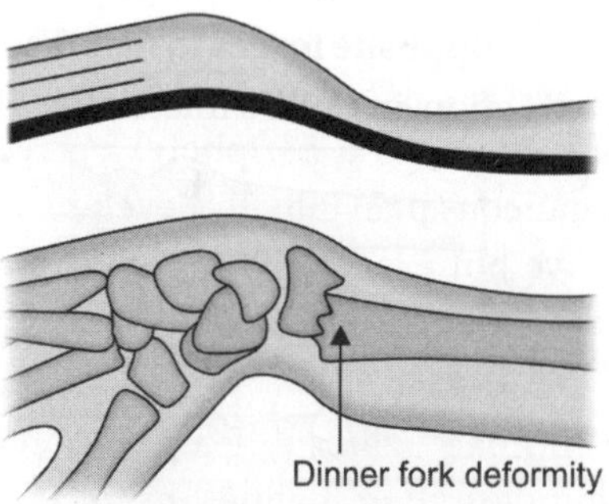

Fig. 7.14: Malunited colles

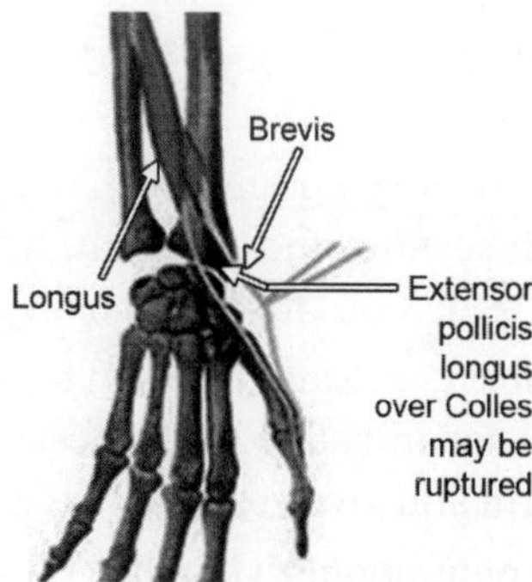

Fig. 7.15: EPL injury

- Carpal tunnel syndrome causing median nerve compression.
- Carpal instability
- Triangular-fibro cartilage complex (TFCC) injury and subluxation of inferior radioulnar joint.
- Delayed union and nonunion are extremely rare.

Smith fracture (reverse Colles fracture). It is an extra-articular fracture of lower end of radius with volar displacement. It is treated by cast (Above elbow) and malunion causes Garden-Spade deformity

SUDECK'S OSTEONEURO DYSTROPHY

Sudeck's osteoneuro dystrophy/reflex sympathetic dystrophy/causalgia/algodystrophy/complex regional pain syndrome

CRPS type I is a regional pain syndrome that usually develops after tissue trauma. The symptoms are unrelated to the severity of the initial trauma and are not confined to the distribution of a single peripheral nerve. CRPS type II is a regional pain syndrome that develops after injury to a peripheral nerve, usually a major nerve trunk. Spontaneous pain initially develops within the territory of the affected nerve but eventually may spread outside the nerve distribution. Median > Sciatic(Tibial trunk) are the most common nerves involved.

Pain is the primary clinical feature of CRPS. Vasomotor dysfunction, sudomotor abnormalities, or focal edema may occur alone or in combination but must be present for diagnosis. In CRPS, localized sweating (increased resting sweat output) and changes in blood flow may produce temperature differences between affected and unaffected limbs.

The most characteristic symptom is pain out of proportion to the inciting event in both severity and duration. It is often burning in character. Hence the term 'Causalgia' which means burning pain.

Swelling is the most consistent physical finding. It often begins in area of injury and is soft initially as the process continues, oedema gradually becomes firm and involves much broader area.

Stiffness and discolouration of skin (red, blue and/or pallor) are other classic signs.

Trophic skin changes i.e. skin is shiny, thin with loss of normal wrinkles and creases are characteristically seen late. **The most common radiographic finding is localized osteopenia**-increased blood flow to the bone Prognosis is directly related to the time to diagnosis and initiation of therapy. The goal is to break abnormal sympathetic Reflex and to restore motion.

Clinical trials suggest that early mobilization with physical therapy or a brief course of glucocorticoids may be helpful for CRPS type I. Other medical treatments include the use of adrenergic blockers, nonsteroidal anti-inflammatory drugs, calcium channel blockers, phenytoin, opioids, and calcitonin. Stellate ganglion blockade is a commonly used invasive therapeutic technique that often provides temporary pain relief, but the efficacy of repetitive blocks is uncertain.

Recovery is prolonged **and** painful both for patient and surgeon. 3 years usually elapse before the bones are remineralized and it is rare that full range of movements returns.

Note: Reflex Sympathetic Dystrophy- Patchy Osteopenia

Hyperparathyroidism- **Generalised** Osteopenia

Tuberculosis- Disuse Osteopenia

Clavicle

- Clavicle is the most common fractured bone (overall) in adults.
- Clavicle is the most common bone fractured during birth.
- Most common part in middle third fracture
- The weakest point of midclavicle is the junction of middle and outer third (i.e. medial 2/3rd and lateral 1/3rd).
- Sling immobilization/Fig. of eight bandage
- Malunion is the most common complication.

Injury	Common Nerve Involvement
Anterior or inferior shoulder dislocation	Axillary, (circumflex humeral) nerve
Fracture surgical neck humerus	Axillary nerve
Fracture shaft hummerus	Radial nerve
Fracture supracondylar humerus	AIN > Median > Radial > Ulnar (AMRU)
Cubitus valgus	Tardy ulnar nerve palsy

Contd...

Contd...

Injury	Common Nerve Involvement
Medial condyle hummers	Ulnar nerve
Monteggia fracture dislocation	Posterior interosseous nerve
Volkman's ischemic contracture	Anterior Interosseous nerve
Lunate dislocation	Median nerve
Hip dislocation	Sciatic nerve
Knee dislocation	C. Peroneal nerve

Axillary nerve injury shows sensory loss around the regimental badge in army called as regimental badge sign.

Relative Incidence of Carpal Bone Fractures Scaphoid > Triquetral >Trapezium

Scaphoid: Middle third (Waist) fractures are most common.

Sign – Tenderness in anatomical snuff box. **Oblique view important for diagnosis.**

MRI can diagnose occult fractures.

Treatment is glass holding cast if does not unite or markedly displaced fracture Headless screw is used.

Scapholunate dissociation ~ Terry Thomas sign ~ David Letterman sign.

Injuries with characteristic deformities:

Deformity	Injury
Flattening of shoulder	Shoulder dislocation (anterior)
Dinner-fork deformity	Colles' fracture
Garden-Spade Deformity	Smith Fracture
Mallet finger	Avulsion of the insertion of the extensor tendon from distal phalanx
Flexion, adduction and internal rotation of the hip	Posterior dislocation of the hip, arthritis
Flexion, abduction, external rotation of the hip	Anterior dislocation of the hip, septic hip synovitis of hip joint/Fluid in Hip joint and Iliotibial **Band Contracture** (Polio)
External rotation of the leg	1. Fracture neck of femur 2. Trochanteric fracture (Lat border of foot touching bed)

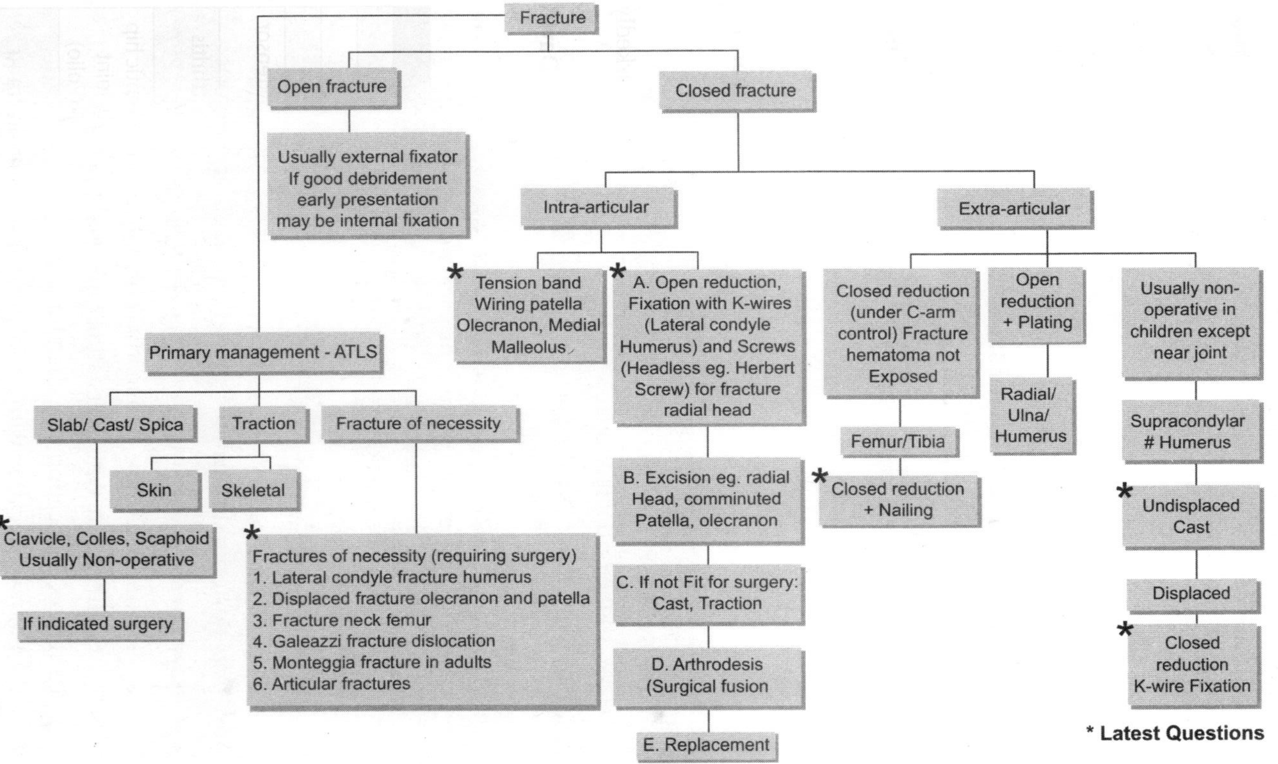
Fracture
Open fracture
Usually external fixator If good debridement early presentation may be internal fixation
Closed fracture
Intra-articular
Extra-articular
* Tension band Wiring patella Olecranon, Medial Malleolus
* A. Open reduction, Fixation with K-wires (Lateral condyle Humerus) and Screws (Headless eg. Herbert Screw) for fracture radial head
B. Excision eg. radial Head, comminuted Patella, olecranon
C. If not Fit for surgery: Cast, Traction
D. Arthrodesis (Surgical fusion
E. Replacement
Closed reduction (under C-arm control) Fracture hematoma not Exposed
Femur/Tibia
* Closed reduction + Nailing
Open reduction + Plating
Radial/ Ulna/ Humerus
Usually non-operative in children except near joint
Supracondylar # Humerus
* Undisplaced Cast
Displaced
* Closed reduction K-wire Fixation
Primary management - ATLS
Slab/ Cast/ Spica
Traction
Fracture of necessity
Skin
Skeletal
* Clavicle, Colles, Scaphoid Usually Non-operative
If indicated surgery
* Fractures of necessity (requiring surgery)
1. Lateral condyle fracture humerus
2. Displaced fracture olecranon and patella
3. Fracture neck femur
4. Galeazzi fracture dislocation
5. Monteggia fracture in adults
6. Articular fractures
* Latest Questions

QUESTIONS

1. **Fracture and dislocation of lateral clavicle. Best treatment is:**
   a. Fig. of 8 splint
   b. Open reduction
   c. Normal sling
   d. Surgical repair

Ans. is 'd' Surgical repair

2. **Mason's classification is used for:**
   a. Clavicle fracture
   b. Colle's fracture
   c. Radial head fracture
   d. Monteggia fracture

Ans. is 'c' Radial head fracture

3. **Muscle in 2nd compartment of wrist:** *(Recent Pattern Question 2018)*
   a. Extensor pollicis brevis
   b. Extensor carpi radialis brevis and longus
   c. Abductor pollicis longus
   d. Extensor pollicis longus

Ans. is 'b' Extensor carpi radialis brevis and longus

4. **A patient received an electric shock and fell down. He cannot do external rotation of shoulder and cannot move arm. What is the diagnosis?** *(Recent Pattern Question 2018)*
   a. Anterior dislocation
   b. Posterior dislocation
   c. Clavicle fracture
   d. Luxation erecta

Ans. is 'b' Posterior dislocation

5. **Terrible triad of elbow is:** *(Recent Pattern Question 2017)*
   a. Humerus fracture with medial epicondyle fracture
   b. Shaft fracture with dislocation and ulnar fracture
   c. Elbow dislocation with shaft fracture
   d. Elbow dislocation with radial head and coronoid fracture

Ans. is 'd' Elbow dislocation with radial head and coronoid fracture

6. **What is true about supracondylar fracture?**
(Recent Pattern Question 2017)
   a. Mostly seen in elderly population
   b. Females are mostly affected
   c. Most common type is extension type
   d. Can cause nonunion

Ans. is 'c' Most common type is extension type

7. **Which of the following is static stabilizer of shoulder joint:**
   a. Supraspinatus
   b. Infraspinatus
   c. Negative pressure in glenoid cavity
   d. Subscapularis

Ans. is 'c' Negative pressure in glenoid cavity

8. **Which of the following test of shoulder dislocation is verified by just looking at the axillary fat folds:**
   a. Dugas test
   b. Callaway test
   c. Hamilton ruler test
   d. Bryants's test

Ans. is 'd' Bryants's test

9. **Colle's fracture which of the following tendons likely to rupture:**
   a. Flexor pollicis longus
   b. Flexor pollicis brevis
   c. Extensor pollicis longus
   d. Extensor pollicis brevis

Ans. is 'c' Extensor pollicis longus

10. **Injury in radial groove of humerus will lead to:**
   a. Wrist drop
   b. Chauffeur's fracture
   c. Skier's thumb
   d. Mallet finger

Ans. is 'a' Wrist drop

11. A 24-year-old sustained the fracture shown in the X-ray below. The nerve most likely to be injured is:

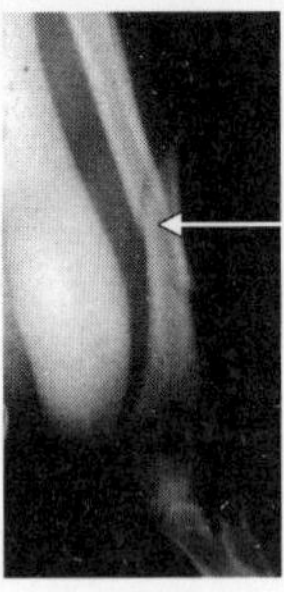

a. Ulnar nerve
b. Medial nerve
c. Radial nerve
d. Musculocutaneous nerve

Ans. is 'c' Radial nerve

12. Eponym for fracture shown in below X-ray is:

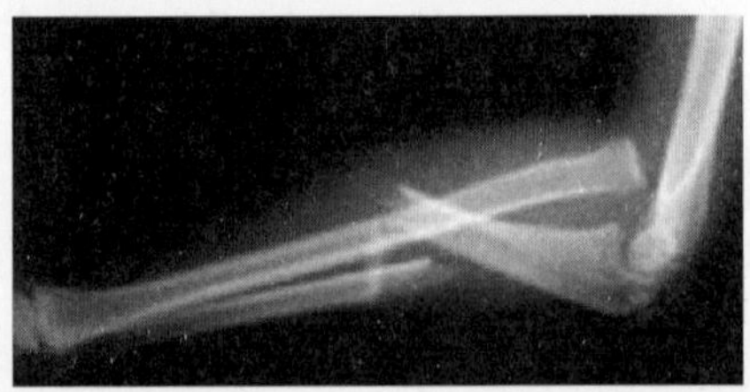

a. Monteggia fracture
b. Colles fracture
c. Galezzei fracture
d. Smith fracture

Ans. is 'a' Monteggia fracture

13. Which nerve is injured in fracture of fibula:

a. Posterior tibial nerve
b. Anterior tibial nerve
c. Common peroneal nerve
d. Deep peroneal nerve

Ans. is 'c' Common peroneal nerve

14. Terry Thomas sign is seen in?

a. Keinbock's disease
b. Carpal instability
c. Calcaneal disorders
d. Hip trauma

Ans. is 'b' Carpal instability

15. Classical sign of scaphoid fracture is?

a. Pain with limited range of motion
b. Pain in snuffbox
c. Scaphoid ring sign
d. Swelling of wrist

Ans. is 'b' Pain in snuffbox

16. Most common fractured bone on face:

a. Nasoethmoid bone
b. Zygomatic bone
c. Nasal bone
d. Mandible

Ans. is 'c' Nasal bone

17. Monteggia fracture is:

a. Fracture of distal radius with dislocation of head of ulna
b. Fracture of the proximal third of the ulna with dislocation of the head of the radius
c. Fracture of distal third of ulna with dislocation of head of radius
d. Fracture of proximal one third of radius with dislocation of head of radius

Ans. is 'b' Fracture of the proximal third of the ulna with dislocation of the head of the radius

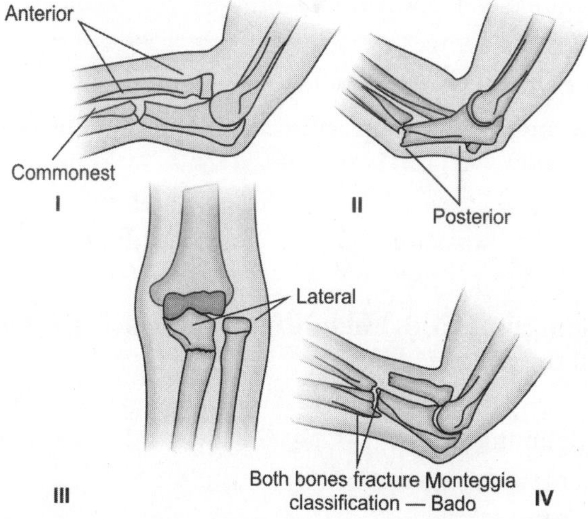

Fig. 7.16: Monteggia fracture—Bado classification

18. Hill-Sach's lesion:

a. Hip joint dislocation b. Elbow dislocation

c. Shoulder dislocation d. Jaw dislocation

Ans. is 'c' Shoulder dislocation

19. First sign of Volkamann's ischemia is:

a. Puseness b. Pallor

c. Paralysis d. Pain

Ans. is 'd' Pain

20. Most common site of fracture of mandible is:

a. Neck of condyle b. Angle of mandible

c. Symphysis d. Ramus

Ans. is 'a' Neck of condyle

21. In Anterior dislocation of shoulder which nerve is commonly affected?

a. Axillary nerve b. Radial nerve

c. Ulnar nerve d. Median nerve

Ans. is 'a' Axillary nerve

22. Supraspinatus injury which of the following is seen:

a. Frozen shoulder

b. Winging of scapula

c. Difficulty in abduction

d. Cannot adduct

Ans. is 'c' Difficulty in abduction

23. In a man lifting up suitcase, posterior dislocation of glenohumeral joint is prevented by:

a. Deltoid b. Latissimus dorsi

c. Anterior constraints d. Short head of biceps

Ans. is 'c' Anterior constraints

24. Patient comes with fracture femur is an acute accident, The 1st thing to do is

a. Secure airway and Treat the shock

b. Splinting

c. Physical examination

d. X-ray

Ans. is 'a' Secure airway and Treat the Shock

25. The commonest type of dislocation of the shoulder is:

a. Anterior
b. Posterior
c. Inferior
d. Superior

Ans. is 'a' Anterior

26. Dugas sign and Hamilton's ruler test are clinical signs which are positive in:

a. Luxation in erecta
b. Anterior dislocation of the hip
c. Posterior dislocation of elbow
d. Anterior dislocation of shoulder

Ans. is 'd' Anterior dislocation of shoulder

27. Bankart's lesion is

a. Avulsion of glenoid labrum
b. Rupture of subscapularis
c. Anterior capsular tear
d. Anterior humeral defect

Ans. is 'a' Avulsion of glenoid labrum

28. Hill-Sachs lesion is seen in: *(March 2005, March 2013 (h))*

a. Recurrent dislocation of elbow
b. Recurrent dislocation of patella
c. Recurrent dislocation of hip
d. Recurrent dislocation of shoulder

Ans. is 'd' Recurrent dislocation of shoulder

29. In which of the following situations is a posterior dislocation of the shoulder more common:

a. Fall on out stretched hand
b. Seat belt injury
c. Grappling injury
d. Following convulsion

Ans. is 'd' Following convulsion

30. Electric Bulb sign seen in

a. Elbow joint dislocation
b. Shoulder joint dislocation
c. Hip joint dislocation
d. All

Ans. is 'b' Shoulder joint dislocation

31. Luxatio erecta is other name of

a. Inferior dislocation of shoulder

b. Posterior dislocation of shoulder

c. Anterior dislocation of shoulder

d. Posterior Lat defect in humeral head

Ans. is 'a' Inferior dislocation of shoulder

32. Nerve commonly injured in anterior dislocation of shoulder joint: *(March 2012)*

a. Radial nerve

b. Circumflex branch of axillary nerve

c. Median nerve

d. Ulnar nerve

Ans. is 'b' Circumflex branch of axillary nerve

33. Axillary nerve injury shows

a. Regimental badge sign b. Foot drop

c. Wrist drop d. Claw hand

e. Erb's palsy

Ans. is 'a' Regimental badge sign

34. Hanging cast is used in the management of:

a. Colle's fracture

b. Humeral shaft fracture

c. Fracture both bone forearm

d. Fracture olecranon

Ans. is 'b' Humerus shaft fracture

35. Nerve involved most commonly in fractures of shaft of humerus is: *(March 2012)*

a. Ulnar nerve b. Musculocutaneous nerve

c. Median nerve d. Radial nerve

Ans. is 'd' Radial nerve

36. First epiphysis to appear around the elbow region is:

a. Head of radius b. Capitulum

c. Trochlea d. Medial condyle

Ans. is 'b' Capitulum

37. 3 Point bony relationship is disturbed in following except:

a. Lateral epicondyle fracture
b. Supracondylar fracture
c. Posterior elbow dislocation
d. Fracture medial epicondyle

Ans. is 'b' Supracondylar fracture

38. The 'three bony point relationship' at the elbow has a lot of clinical significance. Which of the following statements is false

a. In posterior dislocation of elbow the triangle is reversed.
b. In a supracondylar fracture the relationship of the three body points is maintained.
c. The base of the triangle is broadened in inter condylar fracture of humerus.
d. The points are marked out with the elbow in extension

Ans. is 'd' The points are marked out with the elbow in extension

39. Commonest type of supracondylar fracture is the (elbow)

a. Flexion type
b. Extension type
c. Abduction type
d. Subglenoid type

Ans. is 'b' Extension type

40. Humeral supracondylar fracture commonly results in which nerve injury: *(September 2007)*

a. Musculocutaneous nerve
b. Radial nerve
c. Ulnar nerve
d. Median nerve

Ans. is 'd' Median nerve

41. Gun-stock deformity is seen in:

a. Cubitus varus
b. Cubitus valgus
c. Cubitus recurvatus
d. None of the above

Ans. is 'a' Cubitus varus

42. French osteotomy is done for

a. Cubitus valgus
b. Cubitus varus
c. Genu valgum
d. Genu varum

Ans. is 'b' Cubitus varus

43. Tardy ulnar nerve palsy is commonly seen in:

a. Cubitus varus deformity
b. Cubitus valgus deformity
c. Dinner fork deformity
d. Garden spade deformity

Ans. is 'b' Cubitus valgus deformity

44. Complication of humeral lateral epicondyle fracture is: *(September 2008)*

a. Non union
b. Tardy ulnar nerve palsy
c. Cubitus valgus deformity
d. All of the above

Ans. is 'd' All of the above

45. Most common nerve injured in fracture of medial epicondyle of humerus is: *(March 2007)*

a. Radial nerve
b. Ulnar nerve
c. Median nerve
d. Musculocutaneous nerve

Ans. is 'b' Ulnar nerve

46. In Hansen's disease, the nerve commonly affected at elbow is:

a. Ulnar nerve
b. Median nerve
c. Radial nerve
d. Musculocutaneous nerve

Ans. is 'a' Ulnar nerve

47. Compartment syndrome is due to all except

a. Fracture
b. Tight plaster
c. Burns
d. Scorpion bite
e. Snake bite

Ans. is 'd' Scorpion bite

48. Myositis ossificans refers to:

a. Heterotropic bone formation
b. Muscle infection
c. Muscle and bone infection
d. Avulsion of the muscle from the bone

Ans. is 'd' Heterotropic bone formation

49. Treatment of acute myositis ossificans is

a. Immobilization
b. Analgesics
c. Active mobilization
d. Posterior mobilization

Ans. is 'a' Immobilization

50. In VIC, there is maximum involvement of

a. Pronator teres
b. FPL
c. FDS
d. FDP

Ans. is 'd' FDP

51. M/C nerve involvement in VICis

a. Ulnar
b. Post. Interosseous
c. Median
d. Radial

Ans. is 'c' Median

52. Complications of elbow dislocation are all EXCEPT:

a. Vascular injury
b. Median nerve injury
c. Myositis ossificans progressiva
d. VIC

Ans. is 'c' Myositis ossificans progressive

53. While using axillary crutches, elbow should be flexed to: *(March2013 (f))*

a. 10 degrees
b. 20 degrees
c. 30 degrees
d. 40 degrees

Ans. is 'c' 30 degrees

54. True regarding Monteggia fracture is: *(March 2007, March 2013 (a, b, d,f))*

a. Upper ulnar fracture & dislocated radial head
b. Upper radial fracture & dislocated ulna
c. Lower radial fracture & dislocated ulna
d. Lower ulnar fracture & dislocated radius

Ans. is 'a' Upper ulnar fracture & dislocated radial head

55. In Colle's fracture, distal fragment is: *(March 2003)*

a. Shifted dorsally
b. Angulated laterally
c. Supinated
d. All of the above

Ans. is 'd' All of the above

56. All are common displacements after Colles' fracture except:

a. Dorsal displacement
b. Radial shortening
c. Superior radioulnar joint dislocation
d. Impaction

Ans. is 'c' Superior radioulnar joint dislocation

57. Uncommon in Colle's fracture: *(March 2007)*

a. Nonunion
b. Malunion
c. Rupture of EPL tendon
d. Reflex sympathetic dystrophy

Ans. is 'a' Nonunion

58. Following complications occurs commonly in Colle's fracture EXCEPT: *(March 2003)*

a. Malunion
b. Shoulder stiffness
c. Carpal tunnel syndrome
d. Delayed union

Ans. is 'd' Delayed union

59. Dinner fork deformity is seen in:

a. Colles fracture
b. Smith fracture
c. Bartend fracture
d. Chauffeur's fracture

Ans. is 'a' Colles fracture

60. Fracture of distal end of radius may results in loss of function which tendon:

a. Extensor pollicis longus
b. Flexor pollicis brevis
c. Extensor indicis
d. Extensor digitorum

Ans. is 'a' Extensor pollicis longus

61. Sudeck's atrophy is seen in M/C

a. Monteggia fracture
b. Smith fracture
c. Humerus fracture
d. Colles fracture
e. Barton fracture

Ans. is 'd' Colles fracture

62. A lady presents with a history of fracture radius, which was put on plaster of paris cast for 4 wk, after that she developed swelling of hand with shiny skin. what is the most likely diagnosis

a. Rupture of extensor pollicsis longus tendon
b. Myositis ossificans
c. Reflex sympathetic dystrophy
d. Malunion

Ans. is 'c' Reflex sympathetic dystrophy

63. Allen's test is associated with: *(September 2012)*

a. Brachial artery
b. Popliteal artery
c. Dorsalis pedis artery
d. Radial artery

Ans. is 'd' Radial artery

64. The blood supply of the scaphoid is through the

a. Proximal pole
b. Tubercle
c. Waist
d. Distal pole

Ans. is 'd' Distal pole

65. A patient presented with a history of fall on outstretched hand. There is pain & swelling over the radial aspect of the wrist without any obvious deformity. Radial styloid process is at a lower level than the ulnar styloid process. Tenderness can be elicited in anatomical snuff box. Finding are consistent with the diagnosis of: *(March 2013 (e))*

a. Fracture scaphoid
b. Fracture Colle's
c. Fracture pisiform
d. Wrist osteoarthritis

Ans. is 'a' Fracture scaphoid

66. Most common muscle damaged in rotator cuff: *(NEET/DNB Pattern)*

a. Supraspinatus b. Infraspinatus

c. Subscapularis d. Teres minor

Ans. is 'a' Supraspinatus

67. Lift off test is done to assess the function of: *(AI 10)*

a. Supraspinatus b. Infraspinatus

c. Teres minor d. Subscapularis

Ans. is 'd' Subscapularis

68. A person is able to abduct his arm, internally rotate it, place the back of hand on the lumbosacral joint but is not able to lift it from back. What is the Etiology? *(AIIMS Nov 10)*

a. Subscapularis tendon tear

b. Teres major tendon tear

c. Long head of biceps tendon tear

d. Acromioclavicular joint dislocation

Ans. is 'a' Subscapularis tendon tear

69. Most common joint to undergo recurrent dislocation is: *(AI 97, AIIMS 97, NEET/DNB Pattern)*

a. Shoulder joint b. Patella

c. Knee joint d. Hip joint

Ans. is 'a' Shoulder joint

70. Uncomplicated shoulder dislocation most commonly occur in the following direction *(NEET/DNB Pattern)*

a. Anterior b. Posterior

c. Superior d. Medially

Ans. is 'a' Anterior

71. A 20-year-old male presents with anterior shoulder dislocation. This injury is usually caused as a combination of which of the following: *(AIIMS Nov 11)*

a. Abduction & external rotation

b. Adduction & external rotation

c. Abduction & internal rotation

d. Adduction & internal rotation

Ans. is 'a' Abduction & external rotation

72. Anterior dislocation of shoulder is most commonly complicated by: *(PGI 97, AIIMS 95, AI 96 NEET DNB Pattern)*

a. Axillary artery injury
b. Circumflex nerve injury
c. Recurrent dislocation
d. Axillary nerve injury

Ans. is 'c' Circumflex nerve injury

73. Bankart's lesion is seen at: *(AIIMS June 2K)*

a. Post surface of glenoid labrum
b. Ant surface of glenoid labrum
c. Ant part of head of humerus
d. Post part of head of humerus

Ans. is 'b' Ant surface of glenoid labrum

74. A 6-year-old boy has a history of recurrent dislocation of the right shoulder. On examination the orthopedician puts the patient in the supine position and abducts his arm to 90 degrees with the bed as the fulcrum and then externally rotates it but the boy does not allow the test to be performed. The test done by the orthopedician is: *(AIIMS May 01)*

a. Apprehension test
b. Sulcus test
c. Dugas test
d. MC Murray's test

Ans. is 'a' Apprehension test

75. Traumatic glenohumeral instability on one direction with Bankarts lesion are treated by: *(NIMHANS 03)*

a. Conservative methods
b. Surgery
c. Rehabilitation
d. Observation followed by inferior capsule shift

Ans. is 'b' Surgery

76. Posterior glenohumeral instability can be tested by: *(AIIMS May 10. 09)*

a. Jerk test
b. Crank test
c. Fulcrum test
d. Sulcus test

Ans. is 'a' Jerk test

77. The most common bone fractured during birth: *(MP 98)*

a. Clavicle b. Scapula
c. Radius d. Humerus

Ans. is 'a' Clavicle

78. Proximal humerus fracture which has maximum chances of avascular necrosis: *(NEET/DNB Pattern)*

a. One part b. Two part
c. Three part d. Four part

Ans. is 'd' Four part

79. A boy fell down from a tree and has fracture of neck of humerus. He cannot raise his arm because of the Involvement of: *(AI 2K)*

a. Axillary nerve
b. Supraspinatus nerve
c. Musculocutaneous nerve
d. Radial nerve

Ans. is 'a' Axillary nerve

80. All of the following are complications of supracondylar fracture of humerus In children, except: *(AIIMS May 06)*

a. Compartment syndrome
b. Myositis ossificans
c. Malunion
d. Nonunion

Ans. is 'd' Nonunion

81. Volkmann's contracture, which artery is involved: *(NEET/DNB Pattern)*

a. Radial b. Brachial
c. Ulnar d. Interosseus

Ans. is 'b' Brachial

82. Cubitus varus is most commonly seen in: *(AI 94, NEET/DNB Pattern)*

a. Rickets
b. Postinflammatory epiphyseal damage
c. Fracture lateral condyle humerus
d. Malunited supracondylar fracture

Ans. is 'd' Malunited supracondylar fracture

83. Most commonly injured nerve in supracondylar fracture of humerus: *(AI 11)*

a. Median
b. Ulnar
c. Radial
d. Anterior interosseous nerve

Ans. is 'd' Anterior interosseous nerve

84. All of the following are associated with supracondylar fracture of humerus, except: *(AI 02.NEET/DNB Pattern)*

a. It is uncommon after 15 yrs of age
b. Extension type fracture is more common than the flexion type
c. Cubitus varus deformity commonly results following malunion
d. Ulnar nerve is most commonly involved

Ans. is 'd' Ulnar nerve is most commonly involved

85. A 12-year-old child presents with tingling sensation and numbness in the little finger and gives history of fracture in the elbow region 4 years back. The probable fracture is:

a. Lateral condyle fracture humerus
b. Injury to ulnar nerve
c. Supracondylar fracture humerus
d. Dislocation of elbow

Ans. is 'a' Lateral condyle fracture humerus

86. Pulled elbow means: *(NEET/ DNB Pattern)*

a. Fracture of head of radius
b. Subluxation of head of radius
c. Fracture dislocation of elbow
d. Fracture ulna

Ans. is 'b' Subluxation of head of radius

87. A 30 years old male comes to ortho emergency with his 3 years old daughter who is crying. The father gives the history of child being swung by forearm. The most probable diagnosis is: *(AIIMS 01, TN 02)*

a. Supracondylar humerus fracture
b. Elbow dislocation
c. Stress fracture
d. Pulled elbow

Ans. is 'd' Pulled elbow

88. A one and a half year old child holding her father's hand slipped and fell but did not let go of her father's hand. After that she continued to cry and hold the forearm in pronated position and refused to move the affected extremity. Which of the following management of this stage is most appropriate: *(AIIMS Nov 04)*

a. Supinate the forearm
b. Examine the child under GA
c. Elevate the limb and observe
d. Investigate for osteomyelitis

Ans. is 'a' Supinate the forearm

89. Commonest dislocation of elbow: *(NEET/DNB Pattern)*

a. Anterior b. Posterior
c. Both same d. Medial

Ans. is 'b' Posterior

90. Deformity in posterior elbow dislocation: *(NEET/ DNB Pattern)*

a. Flexion b. Extension
c. Both d. None

Ans. is 'a' Flexion

91. An oblique # of olecranon. If displaced proximally. The treatment is: *(AIIMS SP 96)*

a. Excision & resuturing
b. Tension band wiring
c. Elbow is immobilized by cast
d. Open reduction & external fixation

Ans. is 'b' Tension band wiring

92. Fracture of both bone forearm at same level, position of the arm in plaster is: *(AIIMS June 99)*

a. Full supination
b. 10 degree supination
c. Full pronation
d. Mid- prone

Ans. is 'd' Mid- prone

93. Following displacement seen in Colle's fracture EXCEPT: *(AIIMS June 97)*

a. Dorsal tilt
b. Ventral tilt
c. Dorsal displacement
d. Lateral displacement

Ans. is 'b' Ventral tilt

94. Most common complication of Colles #: *(Karn 00, AI 95 97, AIIMS May 95, NEET/DNB Pattern)*

a. Malunion
b. Avascular necrosis
c. Finger stiffness
d. Rupture of EPL tendon

Ans. is 'c' Finger stiffness

95. Dinner fork deformity is seen in: *(NEET/DNB Pattern)*

a. Colle's fracture
b. March fracture
c. Lateral condyle fracture
d. Supracondylar fracture

Ans. is 'a' Colle's fracture

96. Which tendon gets involved in Colle's fracture? *(Rohtak 97, WB 99)*

a. Abductor pollicis longus
b. Extensor pollicis brevis
c. Extensor pollicis longus
d. All the above

Ans. is 'c' Extensor pollicis longus

97. Smith's fracture involves which bone: *(NEET/DNB Pattern)*

a. Distal radius
b. Proximal ulna
c. Metatarsal
d. Patella

Ans. is 'a' Distal radius

98. Most common site of scaphoid fracture is: *(AI 97)*

a. Waist
b. Proximal fragment
c. Distal fragment
d. Tilting of the lunate

Ans. is 'a' Waist

99. In children fracture scaphoid is though rare but usually involves: *(JIPMER 98, AIIMS 92)*

a. Waist
b. Proximal pole
c. Neck
d. Distal pole

Ans. is 'd' Distal pole

100. Which carpal bone fracture causes median nerve involvement? *(NIMS 2000)*

a. Scaphoid
b. Lunate
c. Trapezium
d. Trapezoid

Ans. is 'b' Lunate

101. True regarding mallet finger is: *(AIIMS Nov 00)*

a. Avulsion of tendon at the base of the middle phalanx
b. Avulsion of extensor tendon at the base of the distal phalanx
c. Fracture of distal phalanx
d. Fracture of the proximal phalanx

Ans. is 'b' Avulsion of extensor tendon at the base of the distal phalanx

102. A 30-year-old man involved in a fisticuff, injured his middle finger and noticed slight flexion of DIP joint. X-rays were normal. The most appropriate management at this stage is: *(AIIMS Nov 04)*

a. Ignore
b. Splint the finger in hyperextension
c. Surgical repair of the flexor tendon
d. Buddy strapping

Ans. is 'b' Splint the finger in hyperextension

103. Bennett's fracture is fracture dislocation of base of metacarpal: *(MH 10, PGI 00, UP 88)*

a. 4th
b. 3rd
c. 2nd
d. 1st

Ans. is 'd' 1st

104. Sudeck's dystrophy symptoms are all except:
(NEET/DNB Pattern)

a. Pain
b. Increased bone density
c. Sweating
d. Stiffness

Ans. is 'b' Increased bone density

105. Pollicization can be best described as: *(AI 08)*

a. Toe to thumb transfer
b. Thumb reconstruction
c. Finger shortening
d. Amputation of thumb

Ans. is 'b' Thumb reconstruction

106. Muscle most commonly affected by congenital absence is:
(AI 09)

a. Pectoralis major
b. Semimembranosus
c. Teres minor
d. Gluteus maximus

Ans. is 'a' Pectoralis major

107. Tension band wiring is done in all except:
(NEET/DNB Pattern)

a. Fracture patella
b. Fracture olecranon
c. Fracture medial malleolus
d. Colle's fracture

Ans. is 'b' Colle's fracture

108. The most common cause of Volkmann's ischaemic contracture (V.I.C) in a child is
(PGI 00, AIIMS 99, NEET/DNB Pattern)

a. Intercondylar fracture of humerus
b. Fracture both bone of forearm
c. Fracture lateral condyle of humerus
d. Supracondylar fracture of humerus

Ans. is 'd' Supracondylar fracture of humerus

Chapter 8

Spinal Injury

Vertebroplasty is percutaneous injection of bone cement (PMMA = polymethyl methacrylate) into vertebral body. It can be used for osteolytic spinal metastasis, multiple myeloma, aggressive hemangiomas, vertebral compression fractures (Osteoporotic). Its use is **contraindicated in infections, Tuberculosis.**

Flexion rotation injury is the most common spinal injury

(AIPG 2007)

In axial load injuries (compression injuries), the most common site of trauma is at the thoracolumbar junction

Car seat belt injury causes chance fracture

Burst fracture is a vertical compression fracture.

Jefferson's Fracture—JAT

Jefferson fracture is burst fracture of ring of atlas (C1) vertebrae

Hangman's Fracture

It occurs when a fracture line passes through the neural arch of the axis (C2) vertebrae causing traumatic spondylolisthesis of axis (C2) vertebrae on C3

Note: C1 and C2 injuries usually do not cause neural deficit because of wide spinal canal here.

Areflexic bladder bower and lower limbs

- With symmetrical involvement - Conus medullaris syndrome
- Asymmetrical involvement - Cauda equina syndrome

Cervical spines have highest chances of dislocation without fracture.

Thoracic spine injury has maximum chances of paraplegia

Erichsen's Disease

Railway spine is associated with railway accidents and has some injury mechanism as whiplash injury.

Whiplash Injury

Hyperextension followed by flexion of lower cervical spine

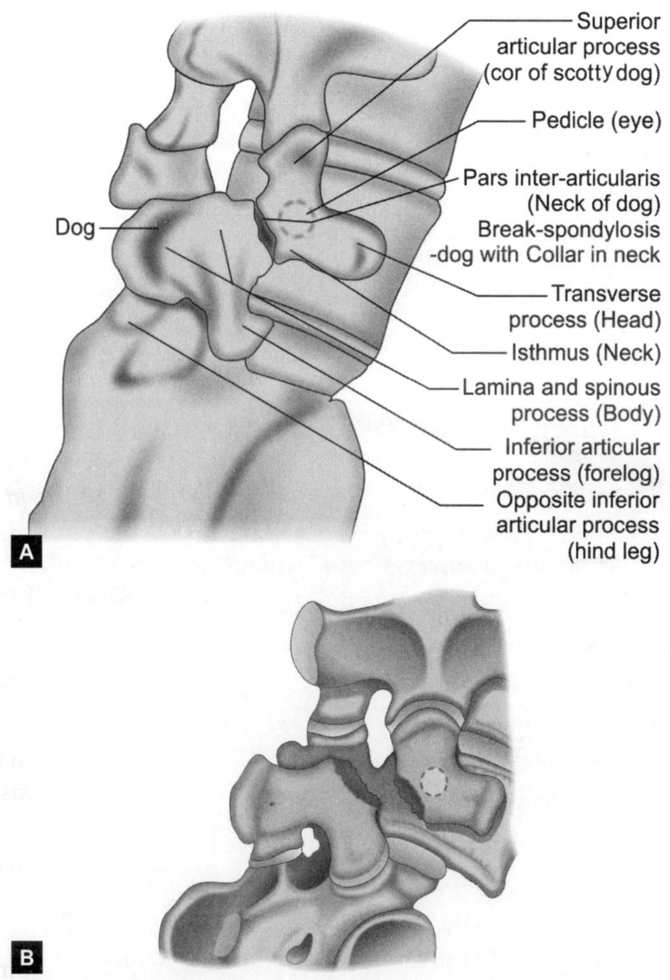

Figs. 8.1A and B: (A) Oblique view of lumbosacral spine; (B) Spondylolisthesis
Slip of one vertebra over other-spondylolisthesis
–Beheaded Dog or Beheaded Scottish Terrier Sign

Scoliosis is Lateral curvature of spine along with rotational component. Cobbs angle is used for its measurement.

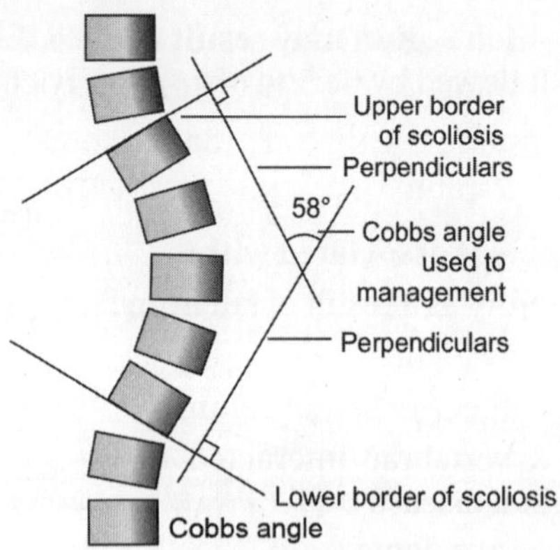

Fig. 8.2: Cobbs angle

QUESTIONS

1. **Jefferson fracture is:** *(Recent Pattern Question 2017)*
   a. C2 fracture
   b. C1 fracture
   c. Fracture of talus
   d. Atlanto-axial dislocation

Ans. is 'b' C1 fracture

2. **Hangman fracture is:** *(Recent Pattern Question 2017)*
   a. C1 ring fracture
   b. C2 odontoid process fracture
   c. C2 pars interarticularis fracture
   d. C7 fracture

Ans. is 'c' C2 pars interarticularis fracture

3. **C6-C7 cervical spine fracture is seen in:**
   a. Chance fracture
   b. Clay-Shoveler's fracture
   c. Hangman's fracture
   d. Jefferson fracture

Ans. is 'b' Clay-Shoveler's fracture

4. **Condition in which there is anterior or posterior displacement of a vertebra in relation to the vertebrae below:**
   a. Spondylosis
   b. Spondylitis
   c. Spondylolisthesis
   d. Spondylolysis

Ans. is 'c' Spondylolisthesis

5. Injury to which region may result in paraplegia:

a. Cervical spine b. Thoracic spine
c. Lumbar spine d. Sacral spine

Ans. is 'b' Thoracic spine

6. Railway spine is associated with: *(March 2013 (d, f, h))*

a. Spine injury as a result of fall from height
b. Railway accidents
c. Lathi charge over spinal column
d. Spine & vertebrae interacted or touched each other in congenital disease

Ans. is 'b' Railway accidents

7. True regarding Hangman's fracture is: *(Manipal 00)*

a. Odontoid process fracture of C2
b. Spondylolisthesis of C2 over C3
c. Whiplash injury
d. Fracture of hyoid bone

Ans. is 'b' Spondylolisthesis of C2 over C3

8. Hangman's fracture is fracture of C2: *(AIIMS 99, AI 93)*

a. Dens fracture b. Lamina
c. Pars interarticularis d. Spinous process

Ans. is 'c' Pars interarticularis

9. Partial anterior dislocation of one segment of the spine over another is: *(NEET/DNB Pattern)*

a. Spondylosis b. Spondylolisthesis
c. Kyphosis d. Scoliosis

Ans. is 'b' Spondylolisthesis

10. In scoliosis degree of deformity is calculated by: *(NEET/DNB Pattern)*

a. Cobbs method b. Hamburger method
c. Raldane method d. Milwaukee method

Ans. is 'a' Cobbs method

11. Jefferson fracture is: *(AIIMS May 95)*

a. Fracture of atlas b. Fracture of axis
c. Fracture of spinous process of C7
d. Fracture of any cervical vertebra

Ans. is 'a' Fracture of atlas

Chapter 9

Pelvis and Hip Injury

Bryant's Triangle: Supratrochanteric

- The patient lies supine and tips of trochanter and ASIS are marked on both sides.
- A perpendicular is dropped from each ASIS on to the bed. From tip of greater trochanter another perpendicular is dropped on to the first one, (base of the triangle). Now join the tips of greater trochanter to ASIS on respective side. Each side of this right angled triangle is compared with its counter part on the normal side.
- Any shortening of the base (i.e. more or less femoral axis continuation line), which may be because of shortening in the neck, head, joint or dislocation of joint can be measured.

TRENDELENBURG SIGN

Normally when the body weight is supported on one limb, the glutei (medius and minimus) of the supported side contract and raise the opposite and unsupported side of pelvis, if the abductor mechanism is defective the unsupported side of pelvis drops and this is known as positive Trendelenburg test.

Trendelenburg test is done to assess the integrity of abductor mechanism. It is positive in the conditions in which any of the three — fulcrum (Femoral Head), lever arm (neck length) or power (muscles/nerve) is affected.

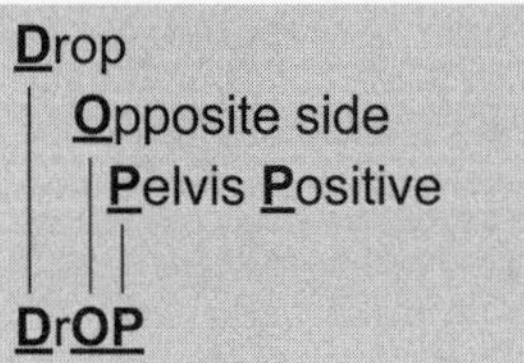

Causes of Positive Trendelenburg Test

Power-Paralysis of abductor muscles

- Superior gluteal nerve palsy (supply gluteus medius and minimus)
- Polio
- Iliotibial tract palsy
- Abductors of hip are - Gluteus medius and minimus (main)
- Tensor fascia lata and sartorius (accessory)

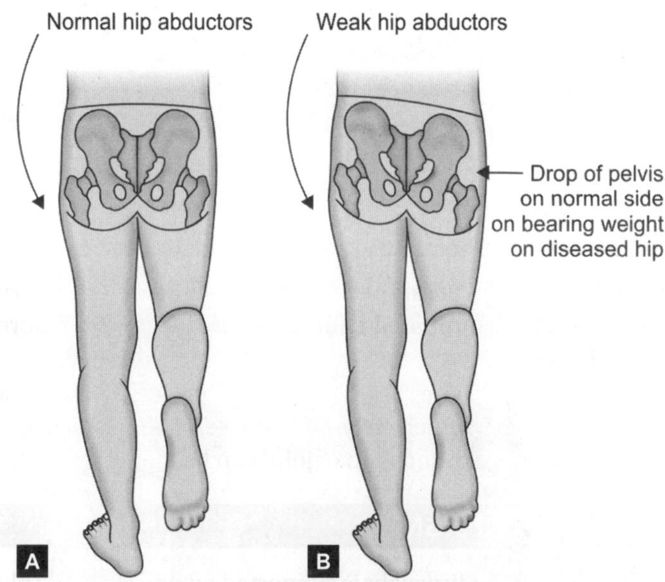

Figs. 9.1A and B: Trendelenburg test

Decreased lever arm

- Fracture neck femur

Absence of stable Fulcrum about which the abductor muscles can act dislocation of hip. Destruction of femoral head as in Perthes disease, AVN, late stages of TB hip (stage 4 and 5) and septic arthritis.

Tuberculosis of Hip- Trendelenberg's test may be positive in TB hip only in late stages (stage 4 and 5) when the head of femur is destroyed.

Patients walk with positive trendelenburg sign on. **One hip-** Lurching/Trendelenburg Gait and **Both hip- Wadding Gait**

Thomas test – to measure fixed flexion deformity of hip by neutralizing lumbar lordosis. **Upto 30 degree flexion deformity of hip can be compensated by lumbar lordosis.**

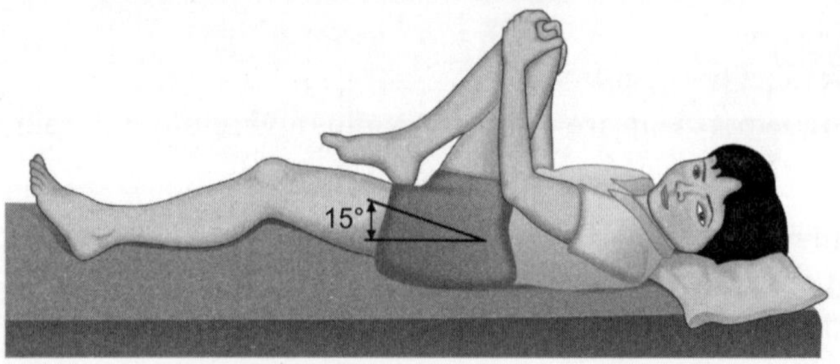

Fig. 9.2: Thomas test to assess hip flexion

Shenton's line is an imaginary semicircular line joining the medial cortex of femoral neck to the lower border of superior pubic ramus. Its femoral part is of more significance. It is breeched in fracture neck femur, head femur, superior pubic rami and dislocation of hip.

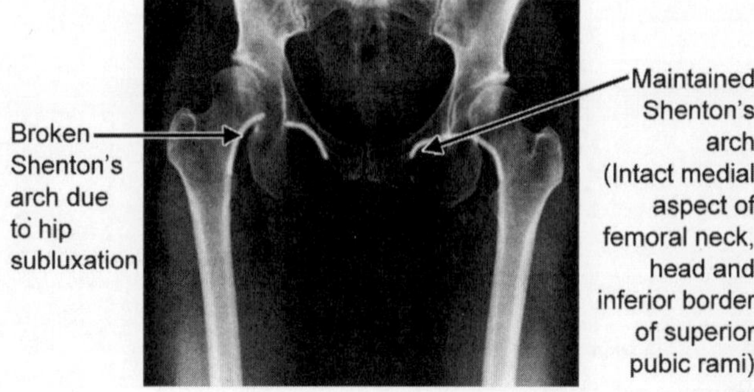

Fig. 9.3: Shenton's arch

FRACTURE AROUND HIP

Deformity of hip

- Flexion, abduction, external rotation, apparent lengthening - Synovitis.
- Flexion, adduction. internal rotation, true shortening—arthritis, posterior dislocation.

- Flexion, abduction, external rotation, true lengthening-anterior dislocation.
- External rotation, shortening-femoral neck fracture.
- Marked external rotation, shortening-intertrochanteric fracture femur.

Fracture Around Hip

MRI is more sensitive (100% sensitivity) and specific for diagnosis of occult fracture neck femur.

Gardens classification is done for fracture neck femur

Pauwel's angle is the angle measured for fracture neck femur and is formed by the line of fracture neck femur with the horizontal plane

Feature	Intracapsular Neck Fracture	Intertrochanteric Fracture more common
Age	Common after 50 yrs (but most common in 7th decade)	Common after 60 years (but most common in 8th decade)
Sex	Both fractures are more common in eld erly females but males are relatively more prone to develop fracture intertrochanteric femur.	
Velocity of trauma	Trivial (usually)	Significant (as compared to neck femur)
Pain	Mild	Severe
Swelling and Ecchymosis	Nil	Severe
Tenderness	In scarpa's triangle	Over greater trochanter
External rotation deformity	<45 degrees	> 45 degrees (lateral border of foot touching couch)
Shortening	<1 inch	>1 inch
Broadening of greater trochanter	Absent	Present
Straight leg raising	May be present in impacted	Absent (Not possible)

Less lateral rotation deformity in fracture neck femur is due to attachment of capsule to the distal fracture fragment.

Fracture Neck of Femur – Treatment

<65 years, ≤3 week:

- **Closed reduction and internal fixation with multiple screw is the treatment of choice. In basicervical fracture Dynamic Hip Screw can be done.**
- **If closed reduction is not possible open reduction and screw fixation is indicated**

<65 years, > 3 week fracture: osteotomy (McMurrays-biomechanical)/ Bone grafting + fixation.

≥65 years

- No pre-existing arthritis – hemiarthroplasty (Austin-Moore prosthesis/thompson prosthesis or modular bipolar prosthesis)
- Pre-existing arthritis—total hip replacement

Complication are Osteonecrosis > Nonunion > arthritis

Chances of AVN and nonunion in decreasing order is

- Subcapital > transcervical >basal >intertrochanteric

Intertrochanteric fracture femur

- Treatment of choice Proximal Femoral Nail > Dynamic Hip Screw
- Most common complication is malunion.

Pelvic Fracture

In pelvis fracture intrapelvic haemorrhage is by far, the most serious complication. Haemorrhage frequently results from fracture surfaces. Amount of blood loss is around 4 – 8 units.

Straddle Fracture

Bilateral fracture of both pubic rami

Hip dislocations: Vascular sign of Narath: Femoral artery pulsations are felt against the femoral head. In posterior dislocation of hip the pulsations are not felt it is called as positive-vascular sign of Narath.

Most common dislocation of hip is posterior.

Associated fracture with dislocations do not have the classical deformities.

Typical/Classical deformities:

1. Flexion Adduction Internal Rotation (FADIR)- Posterior dislocation
2. Flexion Abduction External Rotation (FABER)- Anterior dislocation

3. Central dislocation and Posterior Fracture dislocation (PIPKINS type IV)- Atypical Presentation.

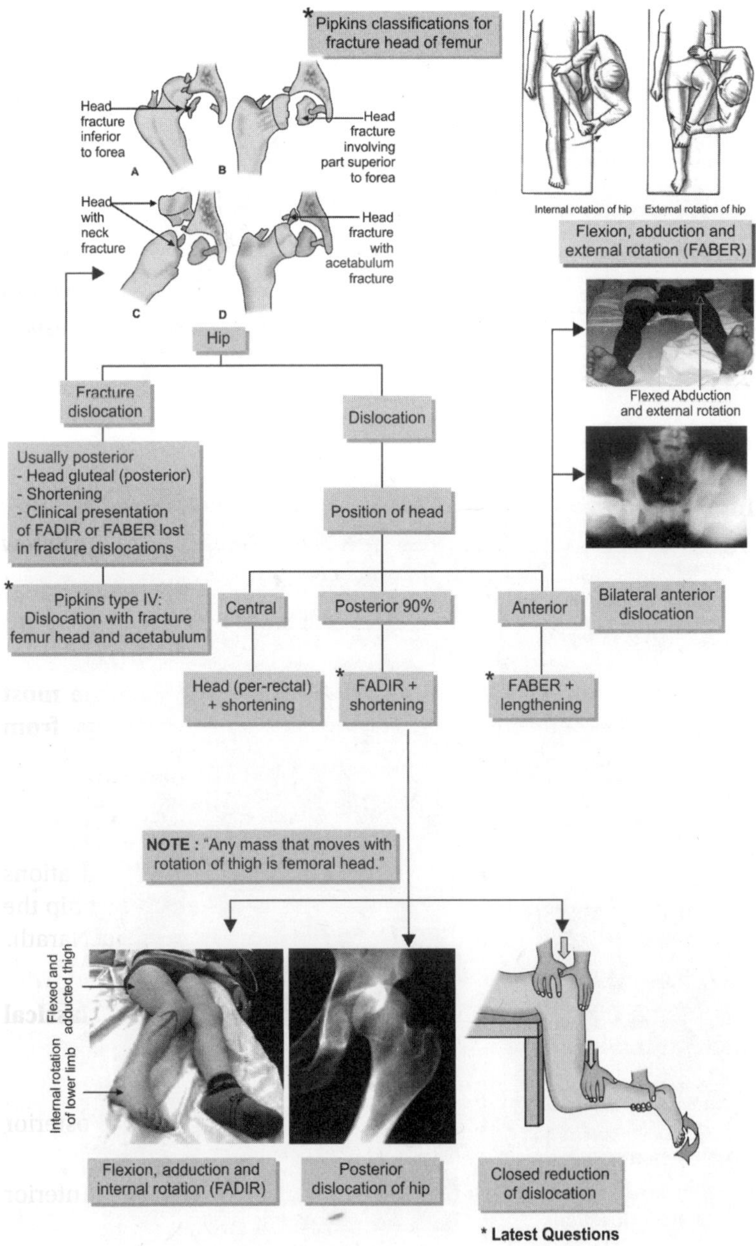

* Latest Questions

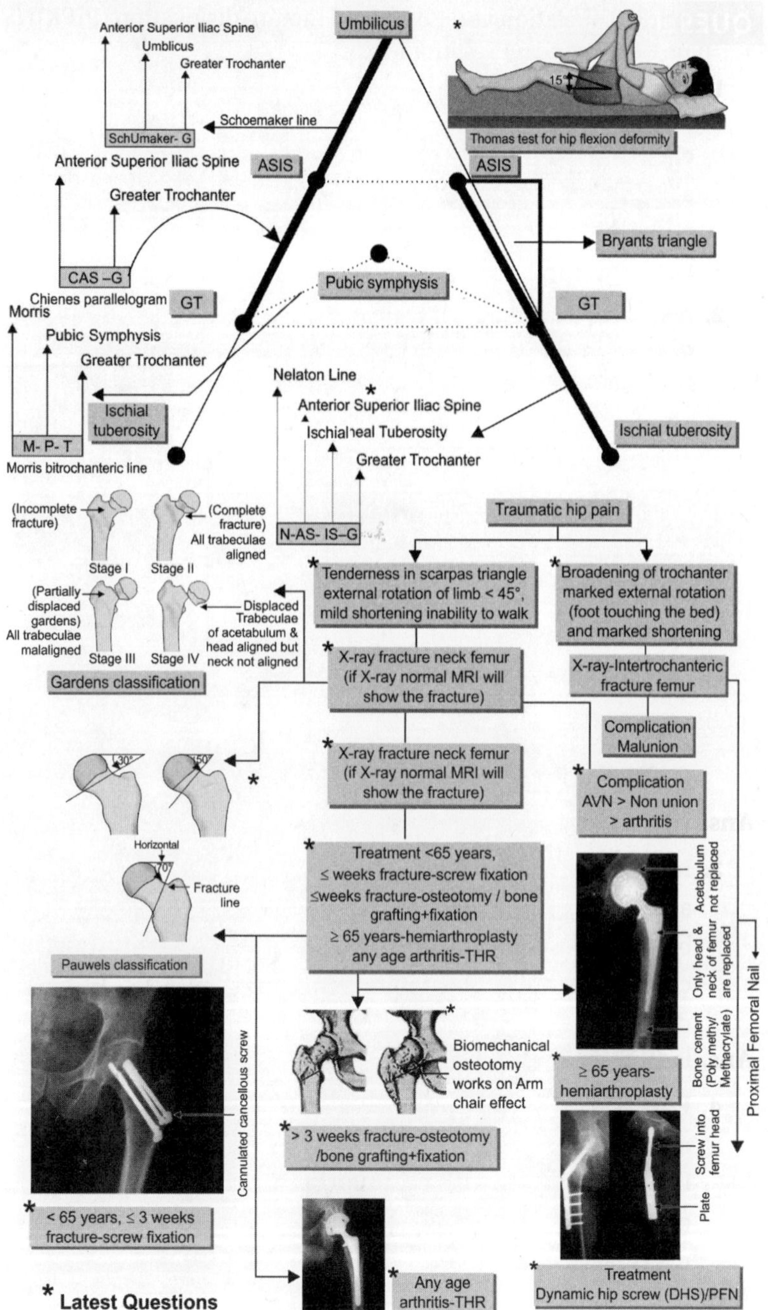

* **Latest Questions**

QUESTIONS

1. **In patient with femoral head fracture associated with femur neck fracture. What is the grading according to pipkin classification:**
   a. Grade I b. Grade II
   c. Grade III d. Grade IV

Ans. is 'c' Grade III

2. **A 30-year-old male fell from a tree. Thereafter he complains of pain and is unable to move his legs (image given). Next management** *(Recent Pattern Question 2016)*

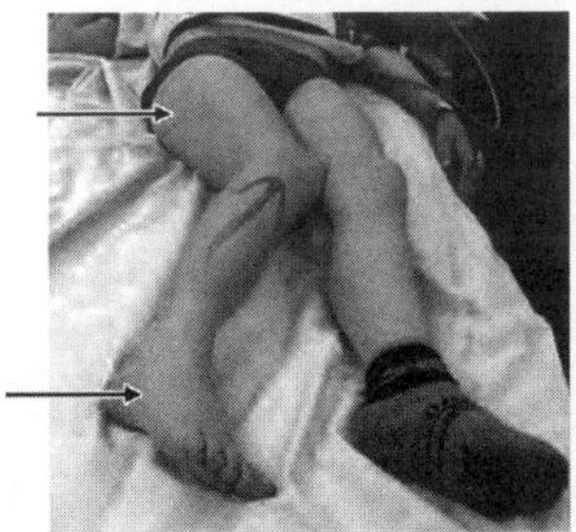

   a. Open reduction b. Urgent closed reduction
   c. Traction d. Observation

Ans. is 'b' Urgent closed reduction

3. **In anterior dislocation of hip, attitude of limb is:**
   a. Flexion, abduction, internal rotation
   b. Flexion, abduction, external rotation
   c. Flexion, adduction, internal rotation
   d. Flexion, adduction, external rotation

Ans. is 'b' Flexion, abduction, external rotation

4. **Postitive trendelenburg's sign is seen in paralysis of?**
   a. Gluteus maximus
   b. Gluteus medius
   c. Calf muscles
   d. Hamstrings

Ans. is 'b' Gluteus medius

5. Posterior dislocation of hip results in:

a. Abduction, internal rotation, extension

b. Adduction, internal rotation, extension

c. Adduction, internal rotation, flexion

d. Abduction, external rotation, flexion

Ans. is 'c' Adduction, internal rotation, flexion

6. Posterio dislocation of hip, which artery pulsations are not felt:

a. Superior gluteal artery b. Inferior gluteal artery

c. Femoral artery d. Obturator artery

Ans. is 'c' Femoral artery

7. Patient came into emergency department with flexion, adduction and internal rotation of hip. Diagnosis?

a. Anterior dislocation of hip

b. Posterior dislocation of hip

c. Central dislocation of hip

d. Fracture neck of femur

Ans. is 'b' Posterior dislocation of hip

8. A 82-year-old female with necrotic head of femur and bilateral osteoarthritis. What is the next step of management:

a. Uncemented total hip replacement

b. Cemented total hip replacement

c. Hemi-arthroplasty

d. Excision Arthroplasty

Ans. is 'b' Cemented total hip replacement

9. Waddling gait due to: *(March 2009)*

a. Bilateral congenital dysplasia of hip

b. Coxa valga

c. CEV

d. Bilateral coxa valgum

Ans. is 'a' Bilateral congenital dysplasia of hip

10. Trendelenburg sign is positive due to the involvement of: *(March 2009)*

a. Gluteum maximus b. Gluteus medius

c. Psoas major d. Adductor magnus

Ans. is 'b' Gluteus medius

11. Trendelenburgs test is positive in injury to: *(September 2012)*

a. Superior gluteal nerve b. Inferior gluteal nerve

c. Pudendal nerve d. Obturator nerve

Ans. is 'a' Superior gluteal nerve

12. Trendelenburg gait is due to paralysis of:

a. Gluteus medius muscle

b. Gluteus minimus muscle

c. Gluteus maximus muscle

d. Quadriceps femoris-muscle

Ans. is 'a' Gluteus medius muscle

13. Bryant's Δ is useful in diagnosis of following except:

a. Supratrochanteric shortening

b. Infratrochanteric shortening

c. Anterior dislocation of hip

d. Posterior dislocation of hip

Ans. is 'b' Infratrochanteric shortening

14. Most common complication following intertrochanteric fracture femur is:

a. Avascular necrosis of femoral head

b. Malunion

c. Rupture of the Iliopsoas tendon

d. Distal gangrene

Ans. is 'b' Malunion

15. Pauwel's classification is used for: *(March 2013 (a))*

a. Fracture scaphoid b. Fracture neck of radius

c. Fracture neck of femur d. Fracture neck of talus

Ans. is 'c' Fracture neck of femur

16. What is the position of the leg in fracture neck of femur:

a. Internal rotation deformity of less than 45 degree
b. External rotation deformity of less than 45 degree
c. Internal rotation deformity of more than 45 degree
d. External rotation deformity of more than 45 degree

Ans. is 'b' External rotation deformity of less than 45 degree

17. Hemireplacement arthroplasty with Austin Moore prosthesis is done for:

a. If patient is > 65 yrs old
b. If patient is < 65 yrs old
c. If fracture is intertrochanteric
d. If fracture is pertrochanteric

Ans. is 'a' If patient is >65 yrs old

18. McMurray"s osteotomy operation is based on the principal of:

a. Mechanical
b. Biological
c. Bio-Mechanical
d. None

Ans. is 'c' Bio-Mechanical

19. Flexion, adduction & internal rotation is characteristic posture in: *(September 2012)*

a. Anterior dislocation of hip joint
b. Posterior dislocation of hip joint
c. Fracture femoral head
d. Fracture shaft femur

Ans. is 'b' Posterior dislocation of hip joint

20. The deformity in posterior dislocation of the hip is:

a. External rotation, extension, adduction
b. External rotation, flexion, adduction
c. Internal rotation, flexion, adduction
d. Internal rotation, extension, adduction

Ans. is 'c' Internal rotation, flexion, adduction

21. Jumper's fracture is seen in: *(PGI 97)*

a. Calcaneum
b. Tibia
c. Pelvis
d. Neck femur

Ans. is 'c' Pelvis

22. Late complication of Acetabular fracture: *(PGI 97)*

a. Avascular necrosis of head of femur
b. Avascular necrosis of lilac crest
c. Fixed deformity of the hip joint
d. Secondary osteoarthritis of hip joint

Ans. is 'd' Secondary osteoarthritis of hip joint

23. An elderly woman was admitted with a fracture of the neck of right femur which failed to unite. On examination an avascular necrosis of the head of femur was noted. The condition would have resulted most probably from the damage to : *(AIIMS Nov 03)*

a. Superior gluteal artery
b. Inferior gluteal artery
c. Acetabular branch of obturator
d. Retinacular branches of circumflex femoral arteries

Ans. is 'd' Retinacular branches of circumflex femoral arteries

24. Main blood supply to the head and neck of femur comes from: *(AI 11)*

a. Lateral circumflex femoral artery
b. Medial circumflex femoral artery
c. Artery of ligamentum teres
d. Popliteal artery

Ans. is 'b' Medial circumflex femoral artery

25. Increase In Pauwel's angle indicates: *(SGPGI 00. MAHE 2K)*

a. Good prognosis
b. Impaction
c. More chances of displacement
d. Trabecular alignment disrupted

Ans. is 'c' More chances of displacement

26. Commonest complication of Trans-cervical fracture of femur is: *(NEET/DNB Pattern)*

a. Nonunion
b. Malunion
c. Avascular necrosis
d. All of the above

Ans. is 'c' Avascular necrosis

27. AVN of femoral head is most common in: *(NEET/DNB Pattern)*

a. Intracapsular fracture neck of femur
b. Extracapsular fracture neck of femur
c. Subtrochanteric fracture
d. Fracture shaft hummers

Ans. is 'a' Intracapsular fracture neck of femur

28. A 50 years male with fracture neck of femur comes after 3 days, treatment of choice is: *(AIIMS June 99)*

a. Hemiarthroplasty
b. Total hip replacement
c. Hip spica
d. CR & IF

Ans. is 'd' CR & IF (Closed reduction and internal fixation)

29. Best treatment for fracture neck femur is a 65 year old lady is: *(AIIMS Dec 94)*

a. POP cast
b. Gleotomy
c. Bone grafting and compression
d. Hemireplacement arthroplasty

Ans. is 'd' Hemireplacement arthroplasty

30. Femoral neck fracture of three weeks old In a young adult should be best treated by one of the following:

a. Total hip replacement
b. Reduction of fracture and femoral osteotomy with head
c. Prosthetic replacement of femoral head
d. Reduction of fracture and multiple pin or screw fixation
e. Upper femoral displacement osteotomy

Ans. is 'd' Reduction of fracture and multiple pin or screw fixation

31. Prosthesis at head of femur applied in: *(UP 98)*

a. 40 years young male with # head of femur
b. 40 years young male with # neck of femur
c. 40 years young male with posterior dislocation of hip
d. 65 years old male with non united fracture neck of femur

Ans. is 'd' 65 years old male with non united fracture neck of femur

32. Most common complication of extra-capsular fracture femur is: *(AI 98)*

a. Malunion
b. Nonunion
c. Osteoarthritis
d. Nerve injury

Ans. is 'a' Malunion

33. A 60 years old man fell In bathroom and was unable to stand, on right buttock region ecchymosis with external rotation of the leg and lateral border of foot touching the bed. The most probable diagnosis is :

a. Extracapsular fracture neck of femur
b. Anterior dislocation of hip
c. Intracapsular fracture neck of femur
d. Posterior dislocation of hip

Ans. is 'a' Extracapsular fracture neck of femur

34. A women aged 60 yrs suffers a fall; her lower limb Is extended and externally rotated; likely diagnosis is: *(AIIMS 98. PGI 95)*

a. Neck of femur #
b. lntertrochanteric femur #
c. Posterior dislocation of hip
d. Anterior dislocation of hip

Ans. is 'a' Neck of femur #

35. Posterior dislocation of hip is characterized by: *(NEET/DNB Pattern)*

a. Marked shortening of limb
b. Lengthening of limb
c. No change in limb length
d. Extension deformity

Ans. is 'a' Marked shortening of limb

36. Sciatic nerve palsy may occur in the following injury: *(NEET/DNB Pattern)*

a. Posterior dislocation of hip joint
b. Fracture neck of femur
c. Trochanteric fracture
d. Anterior dislocation of hip

Ans. is 'a' Posterior dislocation of hip joint

37. Deformity in anterior dislocation of hip is: *(AIIMS Nov 99, DPG 99)*

a. Ext. rotation, abduction, flexion
b. Ext. rotation, adduction, flexion
c. Int. rotation, abduction, flexion
d. Int. rotation, adduction, flexion

Ans. is 'a' Ext. rotation, abduction, flexion

38. Which is true about dislocation of hip joint? *(KA 94)*

a. Posterior dislocation is commoner
b. In posterior dislocation whole lower limb is rotated medially
c. In anterior dislocation whole lower limb is rotated laterally
d. All of the above

Ans. is 'd' All of the above

Chapter 10

Lower Limb Traumatology

FRACTURE SHAFT OF FEMUR

Fractures of the shaft of the femur are among the most common fractures encountered in orthopaedic practice.

Displacements in fracture shaft femur

Proximal Third Fracture

- Proximal fragment flexes, abducts and externally rotates because of gluteus medius and iliopsoas
- Distal fragment is adducted (adductor longus, minimus, magnus and pectineus)

Middle Third Fracture

- Proximal fragments abducts relatively less because of balancing effect of gluteus medius and adductors; but flexion and external rotation by iliopsoas persists.
- Distal fragment is adducted.

Distal Third Fracture

- Proximal Fragment adducts (because adductor over power gluteus medius because of long lever arm). Distal fragment is hyperextended by gastrocnemius.
- **"Lower limb injures associated with maximum shortening are posterior dislocation of hip > fracture shaft femur>Fracture subtrochanteric femur > Intertrochanteric fracture > Fracture Neck Femur."**

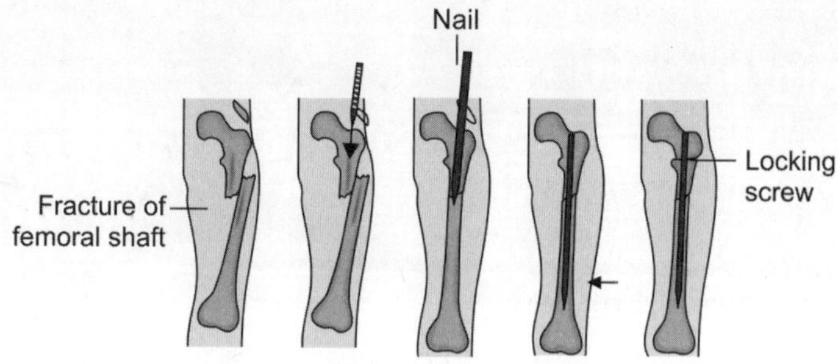

Fig. 10.1: .Closed reduction and internal fixation

Management Plan of Fracture Shaft Femur in Adults

A. Interlock intramedullary nailing currently is considered to be the treatment of choice for most femoral shaft fractures.
B. External fixator is used in open fractures (open injuries)
C. Delayed union is treated by dynamization of nail (removal of proximal or distal screws or both) and bone grafting.
D. Nonunion is treated by exchange nailing (i.e. introduction of large diameter reamed interlocking nail) and bone grafting

Fracture Shaft Femur in Children

Mechanism of Injury: Direct Trauma or Twisting Injury

Most common location: Upper 1/3rd of femur

Management Plan

- Different available modalities of treatment are.
- Gallow traction: <2 years of age and traction weight <2 kg of weight should be used.
- Immediate or early spica casting is the treatment of choice in children <5 years of age for femoral fractures
- Fixation by enders intramedullary flexible rods and plating can be used in children > 6 years of age. It is important to understand that enders nail is more useful in stable fracture pattern and plating in unstable fracture pattern.

Note: Treatment of choice for fracture shaft femur < 5 yrs of age is spica and not gallows traction.

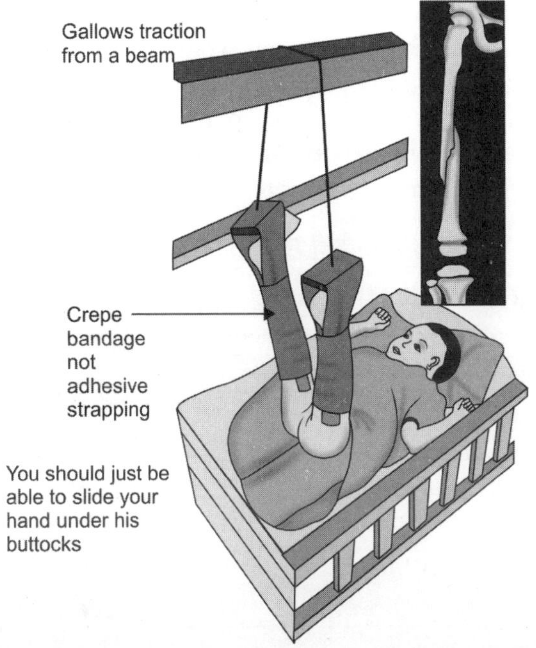

Fig. 10.2: Gallows traction for fracture shaft femur less than 2 years of age

FAT EMBOLISM SYNDROME

Fracture Femur with Breathlessness after 48 hours think of it!

Fat embolism refers to the presence of fat globules in vital organs and peripheral circulation after fracture of a long bone or other major trauma. Fat embolism syndrome reflects a serious systemic manifestation as a consequence to these emboli.

- Fat embolism is a common phenomenon it is more commonly seen in patients with multiple fractures and in fractures involving lower limbs especially femur.
- Fat originates from the site of trauma, particularly from the injured marrow. Fat globules >10 um are considered significant.

Clinical Presentation

- Early warning signs are a **slight rise in temperature and pulse rate (tachycardia)**

The classical triad of fat embolism syndrome is:

1. Respiratory symptoms: Dyspnea or tachypnea.
2. Neurological symptoms: Confusion or disorientation.
3. Petechial rash: In axilla, neck, periumbilical area, conjunctiva of lower lid, front and beck of chest, shoulder.

- Fat embolism is rare in children.

Diagnostic Criterion for Fat Embolism

Gurd's Major Criteria (4)

- Axillary or subconjunctival petechia
- PaO_2 below 60 mmHg
- CNS depression
- Pulmonary oedema

Gurd's Minor Criteria (8)

- Tachycardia
- Fever
- Anemia
- Thrombocytopenia
- Fat globules in sputum
- Fat globules in urine (Gurd Test)
- Increasing ESR
- Retinal emboli
- **1 major + 4 minor = fat embolism**

Prevention

1. Fracture stabilization
2. Removing fat emboli from circulation by:
   a. Lipolytic agents as heparin (increase serum lipase activity).
   b. Hypertonic glucose (decrease FFA production).
3. Offset its effect by:
   a. Dextran (expand plasma volume, reduces RBC aggregation and platelet adherence) .
   b. Aprotinin (protease inhibitor) decreases platelet aggregation and serotonin release.
   c. Alcohol has vasodilator and lipolytic effect.

Treatment

The aim of treatment is maintaining adequate oxygen level in the blood. If necessary by using intermittent positive pressure ventilation. Oxygen is the only therapeutic tool of proven use. It should be administered in sufficient amount to maintain arterial PO_2 >80 mm Hg. O_2 toxicity (pneumonitis) is avoided by using O_2 conc. below 40%.

Steroids are given to avoid pneumonitis.

- Injuries around the knee and fractures of supracondylar can cause damage to popliteal artery.
- Knee effusion is tested by Patellar tap,filling of lateral fossae and fluctuation.
- Patella commonly dislocates laterally
- Patella fractures are treated by Tension band wiring.
- Compartment syndrome of Leg – Test for toe dorsiflexion *(AIIMS Nov 2008)*
- Use of Single Crutch – In the opposite side for Fracture both bone leg and Hip Pathology and elbow flexion with crutch is 30 degrees.
- **Over 90% of ankle ligament injuries (twisted ankle or ankle sprain involve the lateral ligament complex usually the anterior talofibular ligament).**

Tibial Pilon Fracture

The terms tibial plafond fracture, pilon fracture, and distal tibial explosion fracture all have been used to describe intraarticular fractures of the distal tibia.

Fracture Talus-Complications – OA > AVN

- Secondary Osteoarthritis of ankle and/or subtalar joint occurs some years after injury in over 50% of patients. There are several causes: articular damage because of initial trauma, malunion, distortion of articular surface and AVN.
- Avascular necrosis of body, incidence varies with the severity of displacement: in type 1 <10%, in type II~40%, in type III >90% and in type IV 100%

Calcaneum is the most commonly fractured tarsal bone-Tuber angle of Bohler (Tuber-joint angle)–Reduced in fracture calcaneum and Crucial angle of Gissaine- increases in intra-articular fractures.

(AIIMS May 2007, AIPG 2007)

Calcaneum in over 20% of these patients suffer associated injury of spine (most common), pelvis or hip, base of skull and talus.

Angles in Orthopaedics

- Cobb's angle – Scoliosis
- Kite's angle – CTEV
- Meary's angle – Pes cavus
- Hilgenreiner's epiphyseal angle – Congenital coxa vara
- Baumann's angle – Supra condylar fracture
- Alpha angle and beta angle are for DDH.

Chronic ankle instability can be satisfactorily treated by Watson-Jones operation. In which reconstruction of ankle ligaments is carried out.

Watson-Jones is also a lateral approach to the hip joint, which can be used for hip replacement (although rarely as more commonly used approaches are Moore's posterior and Hardinge's antero-lateral approach.) *(AIIMS Nov 2008)*

March fracture involves 2nd metatarsal neck>3rd metatarsal neck

Lisfrancs dislocation involves tarsometatarsal area

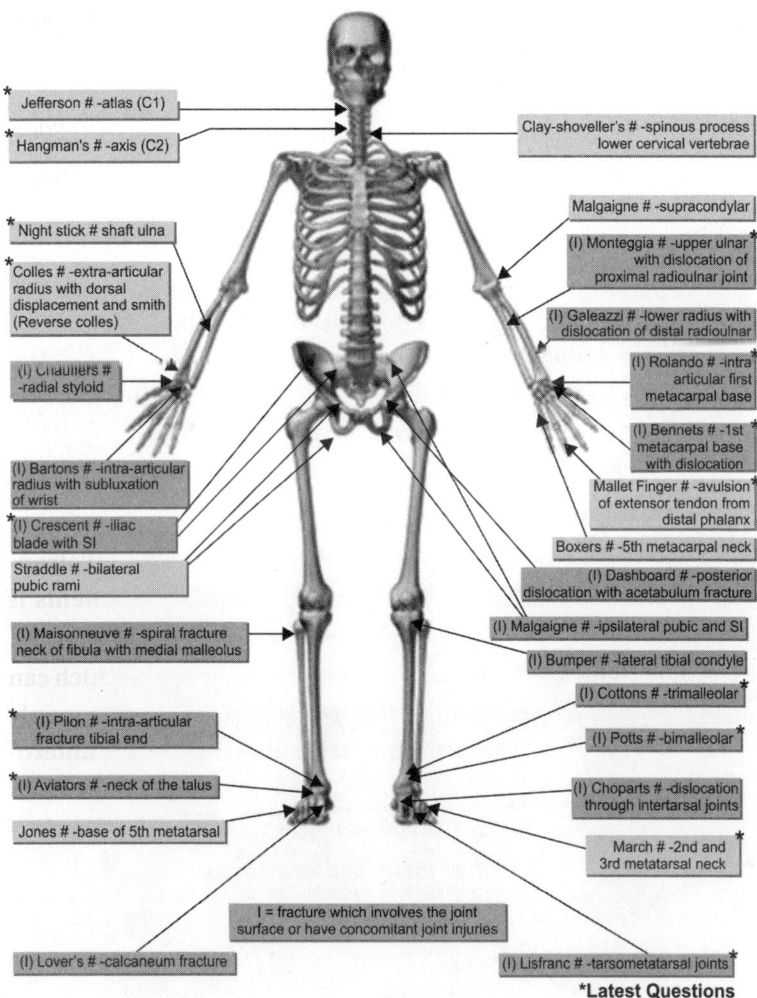
*Jefferson # -atlas (C1)
*Hangman's # -axis (C2)
Clay-shoveller's # -spinous process lower cervical vertebrae
*Night stick # shaft ulna
Malgaigne # -supracondylar
(I) Monteggia # -upper ulnar with dislocation of proximal radioulnar joint*
*Colles # -extra-articular radius with dorsal displacement and smith (Reverse colles)
(I) Galeazzi # -lower radius with dislocation of distal radioulnar
(I) Chauffers # -radial styloid
(I) Rolando # -intra articular first metacarpal base*
(I) Bennets # -1st metacarpal base with dislocation*
(I) Bartons # -intra-articular radius with subluxation of wrist
Mallet Finger # -avulsion of extensor tendon from distal phalanx*
*(I) Crescent # -iliac blade with SI
Boxers # -5th metacarpal neck
Straddle # -bilateral pubic rami
(I) Dashboard # -posterior dislocation with acetabulum fracture
(I) Maisonneuve # -spiral fracture neck of fibula with medial malleolus
(I) Malgaigne # -ipsilateral pubic and SI
(I) Bumper # -lateral tibial condyle
(I) Cottons # -trimalleolar*
*(I) Pilon # -intra-articular fracture tibial end
(I) Potts # -bimalleolar*
*(I) Aviators # -neck of the talus
(I) Choparts # -dislocation through intertarsal joints
Jones # -base of 5th metatarsal
March # -2nd and 3rd metatarsal neck*
I = fracture which involves the joint surface or have concomitant joint injuries
(I) Lover's # -calcaneum fracture
(I) Lisfranc # -tarsometatarsal joints*
*Latest Questions

QUESTIONS

1. **Lauge-Hansen classification belongs to:** *(Recent Pattern Question 2018)*
   a. Femur fracture b. Elbow fracture
   c. Ankle fracture d. Shoulder fracture

Ans. is 'c' Ankle fracture

2. **A patient with fracture of femur shaft develops petechiae, respiratory distress and decreased sPO_2, 5 days after injury. Possible diagnosis is:** *(Recent Pattern Question 2016)*
   a. Hypostatic pneumonia b. Haemolytic anemia
   c. Crush syndrome d. Fat embolism

Ans. is 'd' Fat embolism

3. **Gallow's traction is used for fracture of:**
   a. Neck of femur b. Shaft of femur
   c. Shaft of tibia d. Tibial of plafond

Ans. is 'b' Shaft of femur

4. **Spot diagnosis:**

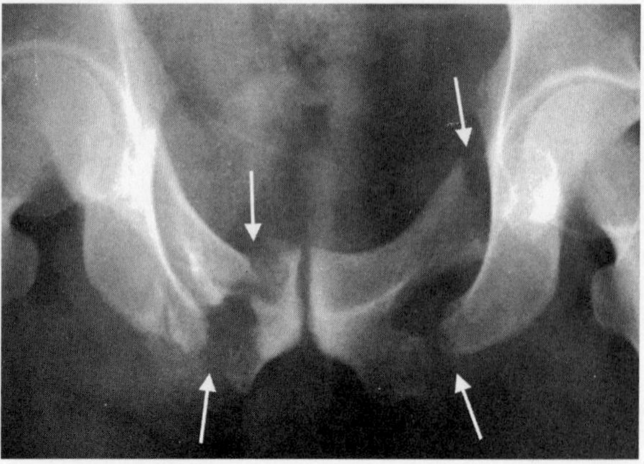

   a. Malgaigne fracture
   b. Straddle fracture
   c. Pubic rami with penile fracture
   d. Sacroiliac joint dislocation only

Ans. is 'b' Straddle fracture

5. Fracture of distal tibial epiphysis with anterolateral displacement is called as?

a. Pott's fracture b. Cotton's fracture
c. Triplane fracture d. Tillaux fracture

Ans. is 'd' Tillaux fracture

6. Hawkin sign denotes?

a. Retained vascularity b. Nonunion
c. Decrease vascularity d. Avascular necrosis

Ans. is 'a' Retained vascularity

7. Stress fracture occurs most commonly in:

a. Metatarsals b. Metacarpals
c. Calcaneum d. Talus

Ans. is 'a' Metatarsals

8. Runners fracture occurs in which bone:

a. Fibula b. Femur
c. Tibia d. All of the above

Ans. is 'a' Fibula

9. Bumper Fracture:

a. Fibula fracture
b. Lateral condyle tibia fracture
c. Medial condyle tibia fracture
d. Femur fracture

Ans. is 'b' Lateral condyle tibia fracture

10. Supracondylar fracture of the femur commonly injures which structure: *(September 2005)*

a. Sciatic nerve b. Popliteal nerve
c. Popliteal vessel d. Femoral vessel

Ans. is 'c' Popliteal vessel

11. Most serious complication of fracture of a long bone is: *(September 2005)*

a. Fat embolism
b. Pulmonary embolism
c. Deep vein thrombosis
d. Associated joint injuries

Ans. is 'a' Fat embolism

12. Effusion in knee is recognized by all of the following EXCEPT:

a. Patellar tap	b. Filling of lateral fossae

c. Patellar shift	d. Fluctuation

Ans. is 'c' Patellar shift

13. Patella commonly dislocates: *(March 2013(h))*

a. Laterally	b. Medially

c. Superiorly	d. Inferiorly

Ans. is 'a' Laterally

14. Lisfranc dislocation:

a. Tarsometatarsal dislocation

b. Lunate dislocation

c. Scaphoid dislocation

d. Posterior dislocation of elbow

Ans. is 'a' Tarsometatarsal dislocation

15. March fracture is fracture of:

a. Calcaneus	b. 2nd metatarsal

c. Distal fibula	d. Proximal tibia

Ans. is 'b' 2nd metatarsal

16. In fracture of femur popliteal artery is common damaged by: *(PGI 93)*

a. Proximal fragment	b. Distal fragment

c. Muscle haematoma	d. Tissue swelling

Ans. is 'b' Distal fragment

17. The traction that Is applied for fracture shaft of the femur In children below 2 years is: *(NEET/DNB Pattern)*

a. Russell's traction	b. Smith's traction

c. Gallow's traction	d. Bryant fraction

Ans. is 'c' Gallow's traction

18. Treatment of displaced transverse fracture of patella: *(PGI June 03, Dec 06)*

a. POP	b. Tension band wiring

c. Screw	d. Patellectomy

Ans. is 'b' Tension band wiring

19. Most common ligament Injured In ankle sprain: *(NEET/DNB Pattern)*

a. Anterior talofibular
b. Posterior talofibular
c. Deltoid
d. Calcaneofibular

Ans. is 'a' Anterior talofibular

20. Bohler's angle Is decreased in fracture of: *(AIIMS May 07, AI 07)*

a. Calcaneum b. Talus
c. Navicular d. Cuboid

Ans. is 'a' Calcaneum

21. Commonest site of fracture leading to fat embolism is: *(AI 99)*

a. Tibia # b. Femur #
c. Humerus # d. Ulna#

Ans. is 'b' Femur #

22. The management of fat embolism includes all of the following except: *(AI 04)*

a. Oxygen
b. Heparinization
c. Low molecular weight dextran
d. Pulmonary embolectomy

Ans. is 'd' Pulmonary embolectomy

23. Recurrent dislocations are least commonly seen in: *(AI 09)*

a. Ankle b. Hip
c. Shoulder d. Patella

Ans. is 'a' Ankle

24. Aviator fracture is: *(COMED 09)*

a. Fracture neck of talus
b. Fracture scaphoid
c. Fracture calcaneum
d. Fracture 5th metatarsal

Ans. is 'a' Fracture neck of talus

25. Tarsometatarsal amputation is also known as:
(KA 99, UP 97, AIMS SR 06)

a. Chopart's amputation
b. Lisfranc amputation
c. Pirogoff amputation
d. Symes amputation

Ans. is 'b' Lisfranc amputation

26. Which of the following Injuries is likely to cause a severe vascular damage? *(NEET/DPB Pattern)*

a. Closed posterior dislocation of knee
b. Elbow dislocation [posterior]
c. Fracture middle 1/3rd of clavicle
d. Tibial plateau fracture

Ans. is 'a' Closed posterior dislocation of knee

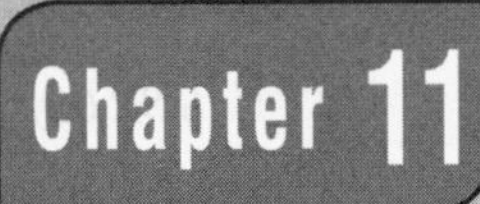

Fracture Management

Common Splints/Braces and Their Uses

Name	Use
• Dennis Brown splint	CTEV
• Cock-up splint (Non dynamic splint)	Radial nerve palsy
• Knuckle bender splint	Ulnar nerve palsy >Median nerve palsy
• Volkmann's splint or Turn Buckle splint	Volkmann's ischemic contracture (VIC)
• Aeroplane splint	Brachial plexus injury
• Lumbar corset	Backache
• Gallows' s traction	Fracture shaft of femur in children below 2 years (or <12kg body weight)
• Dunlop traction	Supracondylar fracture of humerus
• Palvic harness, Von Rosen splint Ilfeld or Craig splint	Developmental Dysplasia of Hip
• Broom stick (Petrie) cast	Legg Calve-Perthes Disease
• Figure of eight bandage	Clavicle

Plaster Casts and Their Uses

Name of the cast	Use
Minerva cast	Cervical spine disease
Risser's cast	Scoliosis

Contd...

Contd…

Name of the cast	Use
Turn-buckle cast	Scoliosis
Shoulder spica*	Shoulder immobilization
U-Slab/hanging cast	Fracture of the humerus
Hip spica	Fracture of the femur
Cylinder cast/tube cast Patellar tendon bearing	Fracture of the patella
cast(PTB cast)	Fracture of the tibia
Colle's cast	Fracture lower end radius
Glass holding cast	Fracture scaphoid[Q]

Gallows traction – Fracture shaft femur < 2 years of age.

Please remember that best treatment for fracture shaft femur <5 years of age is Hip Spica if it is not given as an option than <2 years of age Gallows traction is to be preferred.

(AIIMS May 2012, Nov 2011, Nov 2010)

Skin traction is given through skin maximum weight is 5 Kg and maximum weight of skeletal traction(given through bone) is 20 Kg

External Fixator is Used for Open Fracture

Open reduction is done for lateral condyle fracture humerus.

Tension band wiring is use for fracture patella and olecranon.

K wire is use for circulage and fixation in children.

Upper limb bones (humerus, radius an ulna) plating is done usually.

Lower limb bones (femur and tibia) nailing is done usually.

Ilizarov fixator is used for Shortening with discharging sinus, nonunion and also for CTEV. *(AIIMS Nov 2009)*

Surgical Excision is Never done in growth plate injury e.g. Lateral condyle fracture

Iliac crest is the ideal and most common site for harvesting bone graft. *(AI 2008)*

Iliac crest is the site for 1st order bone grafting

Reimplantation of amputated limb 1st repaired is Bone.

(Skin is preserved 1st)

QUESTIONS

1. The image shows?

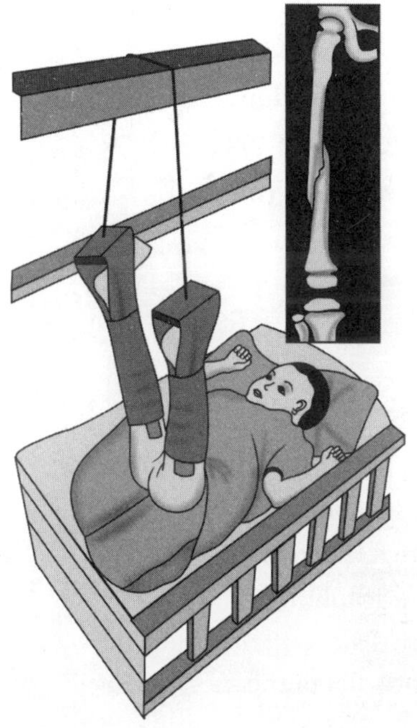

a. Gallow's traction
b. 90–90 traction
c. Russel traction
d. Agnes hunt traction

Ans. is 'a' Gallow's traction

2. Ideal site for bone great harvesting (Treatment):

a. Iliac Crest
b. Skull bone
c. Femur cortex
d. Tibial cortex

Ans. is 'a' Iliac crest

3. Open reduction of children is required for (Treatment):

a. Lateral humeral condyle
b. Femoral condyle
c. Fracture both bone of forearm
d. Distal tibial epiphysis

Ans. is 'a' Lateral humeral condyle

4. Ideal treatment for transverse fracture (displaced) of the patella is:

a. Patellectomy
b. Excision of the lower fragment
c. Tension band wiring
d. POP cast application

Ans. is 'c' Tension band wiring

5. Ideal spare bone of graft is:

a. Tibia
b. Fibulas
c. Iliac crest
d. None

Ans. is 'c' Iliac crest

6. Tension band wiring is best done for:

a. Fracture olecranon
b. Fracture talar body
c. Fracture scaphoid
d. Fracture distal end of radius

Ans. is 'a' Fracture olecranon

7. Maximum weight that can be given with skeletal traction is:

a. 5 kg b. 10 kg
c. 15kg d. 20 kg

Ans. is 'd' 20 kg

8. K-Wire is used in:

a. Cerclage
b. Fixing forearm bone
c. Both
d. None

Ans. is 'c' Both

9. Non Dynamic splint is:

a. Banjo b. Opponons
c. Cock up d. Brand

Ans. is 'c' Cock up

10. Which of the following is the most convenient method for treatment of fracture shaft femur in children less than 2 years of age:

a. Open reduction and internal fixation

b. Reduction and Above Knee POP cast

c. Gallows traction

d. External fixation

Ans. is 'c' Gallows traction

11. Which of the following is ideal site for harvesting bone graft: *(AI 08)*

a. Iliac crest
b. Distal end of the humerus
c. Distal end of femur
d. Fibula

Ans. is 'a' Iliac crest

12. Open fracture is treated by: *(UP 98)*

a. Tourniquet
b. Internal fixation
c. Debridement
d. External fixation

Ans. is 'b' Internal fixation; 'c' Debridement; 'd' External fixation

13. Maximum weight for skin traction: *(NEET/DNB Pattern)*

a. 12 kg
b. 4-5 kg
c. 10-15 kg
d. 15-20 kg

Ans. is 'b' 4-5 kg

14. Tube (Cylinder) cast is applied for the fracture of: *(AI 07)*

a. Shoulder
b. Hip
c. Pelvis
d. Knee

Ans. is 'd' Knee

15. Patellar tendon bearing POP cast is indicated in the following fracture: *(AI 02)*

a. Patella
b. Tibia
c. Medial malleolus
d. Femur

Ans. is 'b' Tibia

Chapter 12

Sports Injury

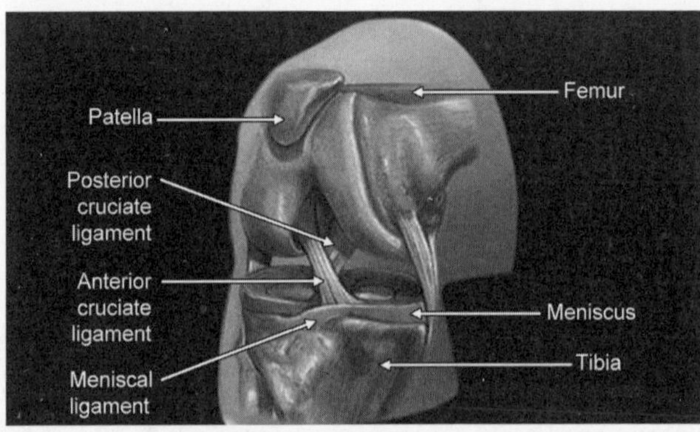

Fig. 12.1: Knee anatomy

ACL	PCL (Stouter Ligamentous Structure)
• It is intracapsular, extrasynovial	• It is intracapsular, extrasynovial
• It is major stabilizer of knee. Its mechanism is to stabilize internal rotation and extension of tibia on femur. Its function is multiple in that it limits forward gliding of tibia on femur and limits hyperextension It makes a significant contribution to lateral stability and limits anterolateral rotation of tibia on femur. It is injured by occurrence of excessive movements which it limits.	• It limits backward glide of tibia on femur (posterior translation) and checks hyperextension only after the ACL is ruptured. • Classically injured by high velocity trauma with posterior dislocation of tibia on a flexed knee as in a 'dash board impact' in a motor car. (Remember Dash Board Injury is posterior dislocation of hip also) Posterior cruciate ligament is active in all knee movements.

Contd...

Contd...

ACL	PCL (Stouter Ligamentous Structure)
• **Anterior Cruciate Ligament:** - Lachman's test (most sensitive done at 20° knee flexion) - Anterior drawer test (done at 90°of knee flexion) - Test for ACL in decreasing order of sensitivity and specificity: - Lachman's test > Flexion rotation drawer test> - Anterior drawer test > pivot shift phenomenon tested by lateral - pivot shift test of macintosh or jerk test of Hughston and loose.	**Posterior Cruciate Ligament** • Posterior tibial sag • Posterior drawer test • Reverse pivot shift test • Quadriceps active test
• Treatment of ACL tear-Arthroscopic ACL reconstruction with hamstring graft (Remember ligaments are usually reconstructed not repaired)	• Treatment is Arthroscopic reconstruction

Lachman's test is the most sensitive test for anterior cruciate ligament tears. It is done with the knee. flexed at 20 degrees. So it can be done in acute as well as chronic injuries. (because in acute cases with hemarthrosis more flexion is usually not possible so performing anterior drawer test is difficult as it is performed in 90 degrees knee flexion).

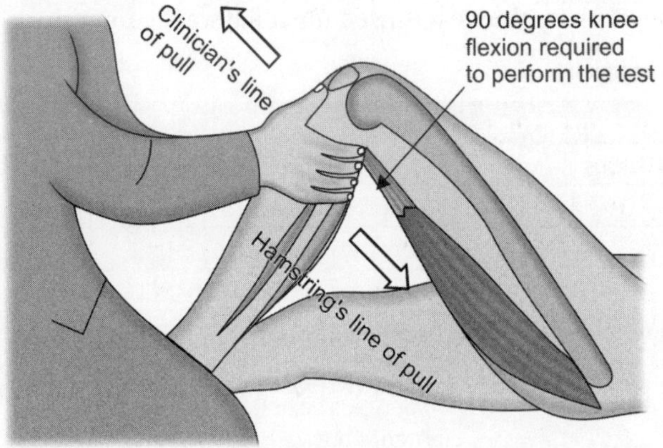

Fig. 12.2: Anterior drawer test

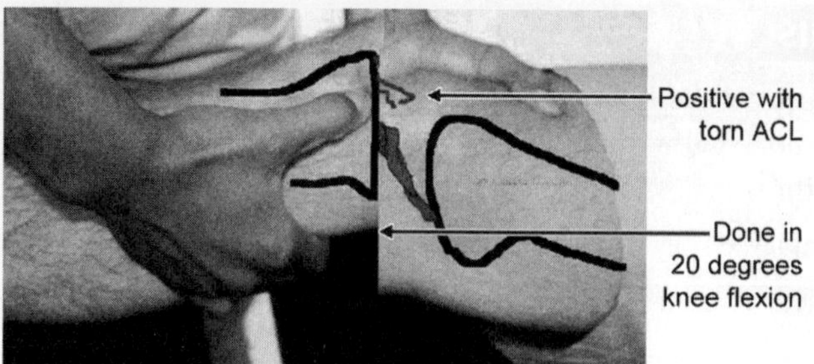

Fig. 12.3: Lachman test

COLLATERAL LIGAMENT INJURY

- The most common mechanism of ligament disruption of knee is abduction (valgus), flexion and internal rotation of femur on tibia which usually occur in sports in which the foot is planted solidly on the ground and leg is twisted by rotating body.
- The medial structures medial (tibial) collateral ligament (MCL) and medial capsular ligament are first to fail, followed by ACL tear, if the force is of sufficient magnitude. The medial meniscus may be trapped between condyles and have a peripheral tear, thus producing **unhappy triad of 0' Donoghue**.
- Main test for MCL (medial collateral ligament) is valgus (abduction) stress in 30° of knee flexion.
- Varus (Adduction) stress test in 30 degrees flexion (removes the lateral stabilizing effect of iliotibial band so that the lateral collateral ligament can exclusively be examined).
- Apleys distraction test is used for collateral ligaments.

Examination

Direction of force	Position of knee	Ligament tested
Varus/Valgus	Full extension	PCL, Posterior capsule
Varus	30 degrees flexion	LCL
Valgus	30 degrees flexion	MCL
Posterior	90 degrees flexion	PCL
Anterior	30 degrees flexion (Lachman's test)	ACL
	90 degrees flexion (anterior drawer)	ACL
Treatment of collateral ligaments is repair/reconstruction		

MENISCAL INJURY

- The twisting force (rotation) in a weight bearing flexed knee is the commonest mode of meniscal (semilunar cartilage) injury. Medial meniscus > Lateral meniscus. *(AIPG 2010)*

Medial meniscus is more frequently torn than the lateral

Medial Meniscus	Lateral Meniscus
Semilunar in shape (less circular)	Semicircular in shape (C shaped; more circular)
Entire periphery of the meniscus is attached to the joint capsule	Entire periphery of meniscus is not attached to joint capsule (Area where the popliteus tendon crosses the joint through the popliteus hiatus is not attached)
Is attached to the medial collateral ligament	Is not attached to the lateral collateral ligament
Less mobile (due to firmer attachment with joint capsule and medial collateral ligament)	More mobile (due to gaps in attachment with joint capsule and lateral collateral ligament)
More prone to injury (due to reduced mobility) The medial meniscus is three to four times more prone to injury than the lateral meniscus	Less prone to injury (due to increased mobility)

Note: Popliteus muscle sends few fibers into the posterior margin of lateral meniscus. Thus muscle contraction withdraws and protects the lateral meniscus by drawing it posterolaterally during flexion of the knee and medial rotation of the tibia. In meniscus or cruciate tear this change does not take place.

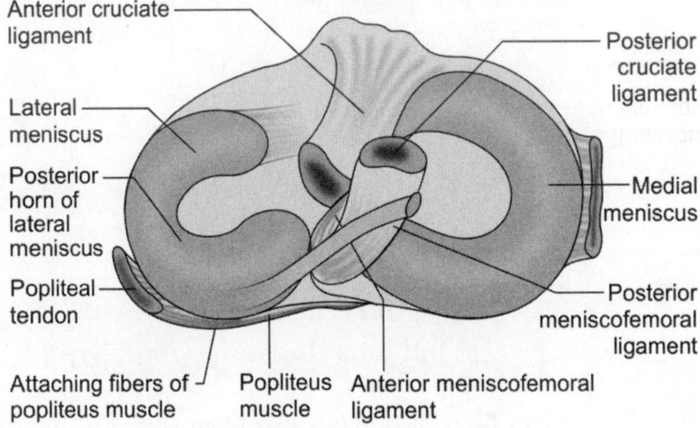

Fig. 12.4: Knee

Meniscal Injury	Cruciate Injury/Collateral Ligament
• Effusion	• Hemarthrosis
• Delayed swelling	• Immediate swelling

Injury to Meniscus

The commonest type of medial meniscal injury in a young adult is the bucket handle tear. **This is vertical longitudinal tear that is complete.**

Smillie Classification – Meniscus Injury

- Symptoms include joint line pain, catching, popping and locking, usually and weakness and giving way (instability) sometimes. Deep squatting and duck walking are usually painful.
  1. McMurray's test is positive
  2. Apley's grinding test is positive
  3. Difficult to perform full squatting and Toe walk in squatting position (Payr's sign)

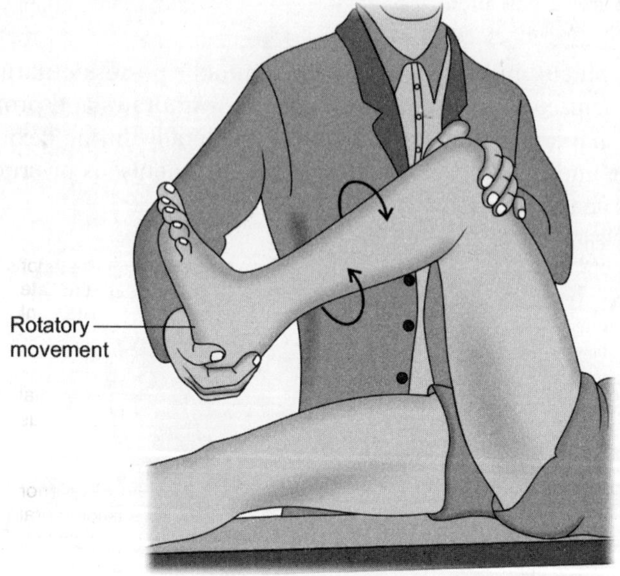

Fig. 12.5: McMurray's test - menisci

Meniscal Injury

- At birth entire meniscus is vascular, decrease in vascularity continues upto age 9 years, when the meniscus closely resembles the adult meniscus. In adults, only 10- 25% of lateral meniscus and 10- 30% of medial meniscus is vascular.
- **Red (Vascular) periphery of menisci**
- **Red- White (border of vascular and avascular area)**
- **White (avascular area) inner 2/3rd of menisci**
- Because of the avascular nature of inner two thirds of the meniscus; cell nutrition is believed to occur mainly through diffusion or mechanical pumping, Inner avascular Meniscus once torn does not heal and requires removal of torn part.
- Tears in the peripheral third of the meniscus, if small (<15 mm), may heal spontaneously because this portion in adults has good blood supply. Larger tears require repair.
- Arthroscopy is the gold standard for making diagnosis and arthroscopic repair or removal.
  1. Meniscal cysts- Lateral > Medial and Pirani Sign- Cysts disappear within joint on flexion
  2. Discoid Meniscus - Lateral > Medial

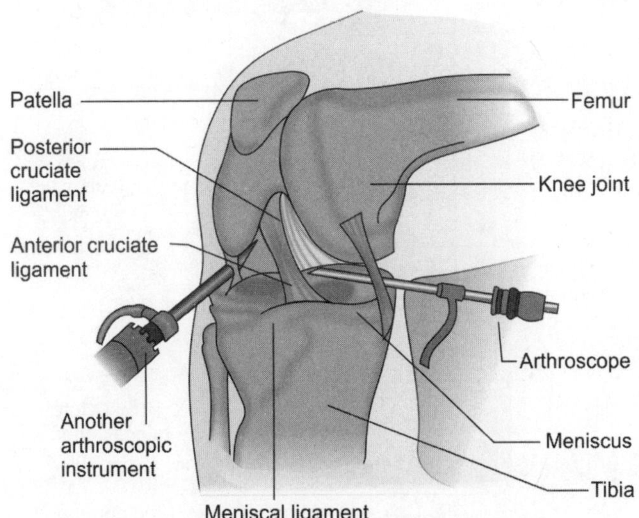

Fig. 12.6: Arthroscopy gold standard for diagnosis and management of most knee injuries

ANKLE LIGAMENT INJURY

Ankle ligamentous injuries, as classified by O'Donoghue, occur as minor ligamentous "stretch" injuries (type I sprain), incomplete ligamentous tears (type II sprain), or complete disruption of the ligament or ligaments (type III sprain).

- The most common site of ligament injury is ankle joint.
- The most common mode of ankle injury is inversion of plantar flexed foot.
- Over 90% of the ankle ligament injury involves lateral collateral ligament usually the anterior talofibular ligament.

Sprains are Treated Initially with

- **Protection** – use crutches to aid walking and minimize further tissue damage
- **Rest** – to minimize further tissue damage and facilitate healing
- **Ice** – to reduce swelling and provide pain relief
- **Compression** – to reduce swelling
- **Elevation** – to reduce swelling

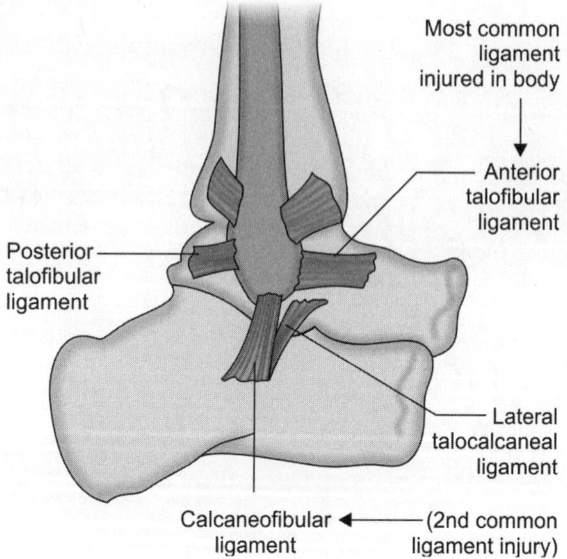

Fig. 12.7: Ligaments around ankle

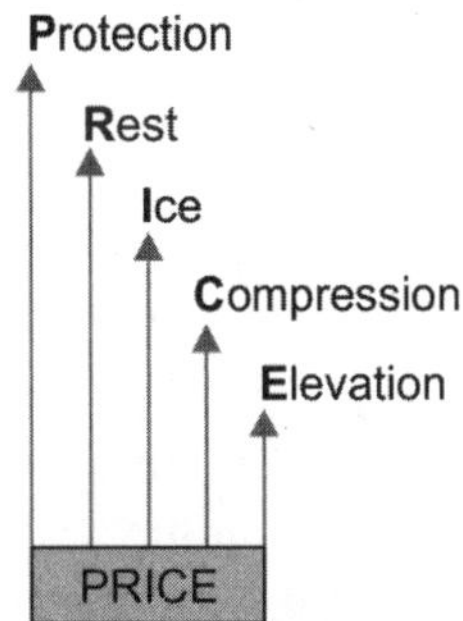

MALLET FINGER/ BASEBALL FINGER

It is avulsion of extensor tendon of the distal interphalangeal joint from its insertion at the base of distal phalanx.

Cause

It may be due to direct trauma, but more often occurs when the finger tip is forcibly bent during active extension (i.e. sudden occurrence of passive flexion of distal interphalangeal joint).

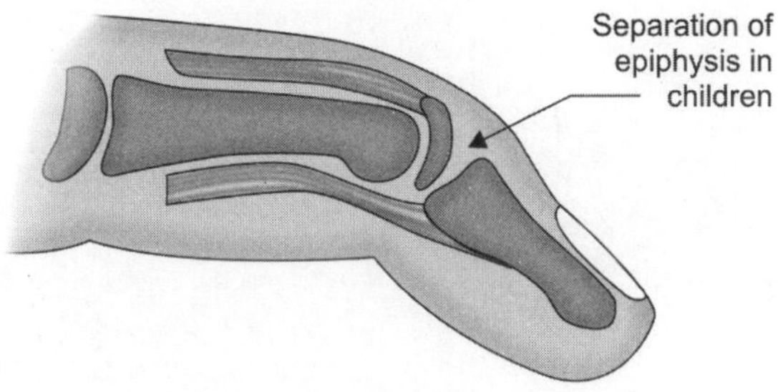

Fig. 12.8: Mallet finger

Presentation and Type

- The terminal phalanx is held flexed and patient cannot straighten it, but passive movement is normal.
- The proximal inter phalangeal joint may become hyper extended due to unbalanced extensor mechanism.
- Three types are a tendinous avulsion (x ray is normal), a small flake of bone or a large dorsal bone fragment, (sometimes with subluxation of Joints).

Treatment

- An acute mallet finger should be splinted and the DIP joint is kept in hyperextension for 8 weeks.
- The twisting force (rotation) in a weight bearing flexed knee is the commonest mode of meniscal (semilunar cartilage) injury. Medial meniscus > Lateral meniscus. *(AIPG 2010)*
- The commonest type of medial meniscal injury in a young adult is the bucket handle tear. This is vertical longitudinal tear that is complete and causes locking of knee

Game Keeper's/ Skier's - Thumb: Injury to the thumb metacarpophalangeal joint ulnar collateral ligament. Due to forced radial deviatory of thumb. Steners lesion is associated. (Trapped adductor pollicis between torn ulnar collateral ligament) Treatment is cast for 4 weeks and if steners lesion is present then surgery.

Mallet finger is avulsion of extensor tendon from the base of distal phalanx and it is treated by Mallet splint for 6 to 8 weeks.

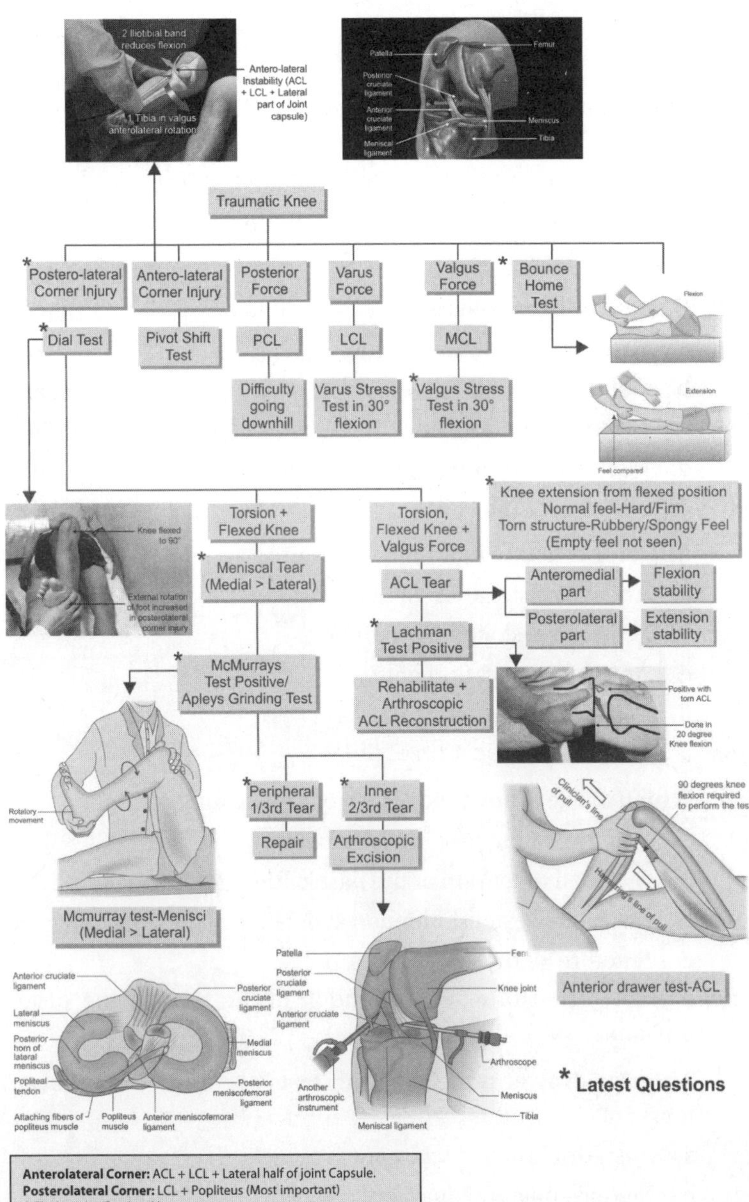

Anterolateral Corner: ACL + LCL + Lateral half of joint Capsule.
Posterolateral Corner: LCL + Popliteus (Most important)
ACL: Anterior Cruciate Ligament
PCL: Posterior Cruciate Ligament
LCL: Lateral Collateral Ligament
MCL: Medial Collateral Ligament

QUESTIONS

1. The ligaments connecting the menisci to the tibia are known as:

a. Coronary
b. Arcuate
c. Transverse
d. Oblique

Ans. is 'a' Coronary

2. Q angle is increased in:

a. Patellar subluxation
b. Genu varum
c. Femoral ante-flexion
d. Medial positioning tibial tuberosity

Ans. is 'a' Patellar subluxation

3. Anterior cruciate ligaments prevents:

a. Anterior dislocation of ulna
b. Posterior dislocation of ulna
c. Anterior dislocation of tibia
d. Posterior dislocation of tibia

Ans. is 'c' Anterior dislocation of tibia

4. Which of the following is true regarding mallet finger:

a. Fracture of the proximal phalanx
b. Avulsion of tendon at the base of the middle phalanx
c. Avulsion of extensor tendon at the base of the distal phalanx
d. Fracture of the distal phalanx

Ans. is 'c' Avulsion of extensor tendon at the base of the distal phalanx

5. Anterior drawer and Lachman tests are done to diagnose tears in:

a. Posterior cruciate ligament
b. Medial collateral ligament
c. Lateral collateral ligament
d. Anterior cruciate ligament

Ans. is 'd' Anterior cruciate ligament

6. The McMurray's test is used in evaluation of

a. Meniscal injuries
b. Fracture of hip
c. A joint following replacement arthroplasty
d. An orthopaedic implant

Ans. is 'a' Meniscal injuries

7. In meniscus injury, 'Locking'-that is sudden inability to extend the knee fully is a feature of:

a. Bucket handle tear
b. Anterior horn tear
c. Posterior horn tear
d. Horizontal tears

Ans. is 'a' Bucket handle tear

8. Manoeuvre carried out for diagnosing medial meniscus injury is: *(March 2010, March 2013 (c, d)*

a. McMurray's test
b. Lachman's test
c. Valgus stress test
d. Varus stress test

Ans. is 'a' McMurray's test

9. Manoeuvre for diagnosing rupture of medial collateral ligament is: *(March 2010)*

a. Posterior drawer test
b. Anterior drawer test
c. Lachman's test
d. Valgus stress test

Ans. is 'd' Valgus stress test

10. The blood supply of anterior cruciate ligament (ACL) is primarily derived from: *(AI 08)*

a. Superior medial genicular artery
b. Descending genicular artery
c. Middle genicular artery
d. Circumflex fibular artery

Ans. is 'c' Middle genicular artery

11. In anterior cruciate ligament tear, which of these tests are positive: *(PGI June 02)*

a. Lachman test
b. McMurray's test
c. Anterior drawer test
d. Posterior drawer test
e. Apley's test

Ans. is 'a' Lachman test, 'c' Anterior drawer test

12. What would be the most reliable test for an acutely injured knee of a 27 year old athlete: *(AIIMS May 02, Jipmer 02)*

a. Anterior drawer test b. Posterior drawer test

c. Lachman test d. Steinmann test

Ans. is 'c' Lachman test

13. Which of the following is the SAFEST test to be performed in a patient with acutely Injured knee joint: *(AI 08)*

a. Lachman test b. Pivot shift test

c. McMurray's test d. Apley's grinding test

Ans. is 'a' Lachman test

14. Which one of the following tests will you adopt while examining a knee joint where you suspect an old tear of anterior cruciate ligament: *(AI 03)*

a. Posterior drawer test b. McMurray test

c. Lachman test d. Pivot shift test

Ans. is 'c' Lachman test

15. Medial meniscus of knee joint is injured more often than the lateral meniscus because the medial meniscus is relatively: *(AIIMS Nov 02)*

a. More mobile b. Less mobile

c. Thinner d. Attached lightly to femur

Ans. is 'b' Less mobile

16. Which type of injury causes more damage to the semi-lunar cartilage In the knee: *(AI 96, AP 99, Jipmer 11)*

a. Flexion and extension at the ankle

b. Rotation on a flexed knee

c. Rotation on an extended knee

d. Squatting position

Ans. is 'b' Rotation on a flexed knee

17. Athletic sustained an injury around the knee joint suspecting cartilage damage, which of the following is an investigation of choice: *(AP 2K. AIIMS 94)*

a. Pain X-ray b. Clinical examination

c. Arthroscopy d. Arthrotomy

Ans. is 'c' Arthroscopy

18. In which of the following meniscal tears will meniscectomy be a more suitable option than meniscal repair? *(AI 08)*

a. Tears in the outer zone

b. Tears in the middle zone

c. Tears in the inner zone

d. Tears at the junction of anterior horn of medial meniscus & tibial collateral ligament

Ans. is 'c' Tears in the inner zone

Chapter 13

Neuromuscular Disease

DISC PROLAPSE

The commonest site of disc prolapse is lumbar spine as here disc are dehydrated. In more than 95% of cases lumbar disc herniation are localized at L_{4-5} (50% cases) and L_5 - S_1 (45% cases). The next commonest site of intervertebral disc prolapse is lower cervical spine (C_{5-6})

Neurological Involvement: Usually lower nerve root is compressed

- Lower nerve root is affected usually like in L4 -5 disc prolapse L5 nerve root is affected.
- **L_5 nerve root supplies Extensor Hallucis longus, thigh abductors, ankle dorsiflexion and sensory supply to lateral aspect of leg dorsum of foot and great toe.** (It is most commonly involved in PIVD L_{4-5}) *(AIIMS May 2012, Nov 2011)*
- S_1 nerve root supplies Flexor hallucis longus, ankle plantar flexion, hip extension and sensation on sole of foot.

LUMBAR DISC HERNIATION

Clinical Presentation

May occur at any age but is most commonly seen at age group 20–40 years uncommon in very young and very old. Typically patient has, Sciatica (pain in back radiating to lower limb) commonly preceded by back pain. Both backache and sciatica are made worse by coughing, straining, sneezing or Valsalva's manoeuvre and prolonged sitting. Standing and supine position reduces pain.

The patient usually stands with slight tilt (list) to one side (sciatic scolioisis). If the disc protrudes medial to the nerve root the tilt is towards the painful side (to relieve pressure on the root) with the far lateral prolapse the tilt is away from painful side.

Straight leg raising (SLR) is restricted (normal is upto 90 degrees).

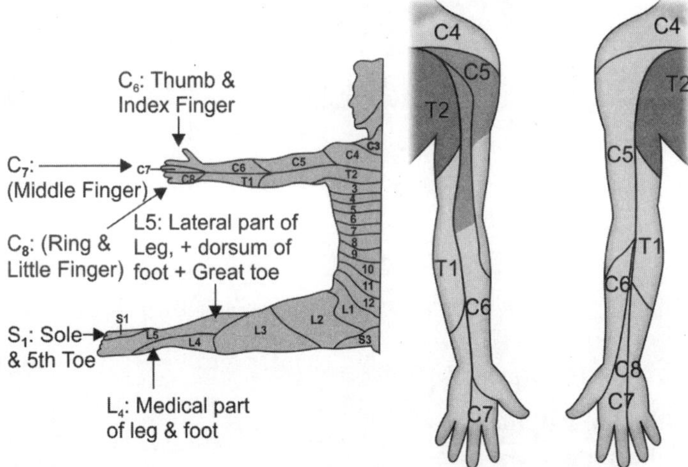

Fig. 13.1: Dermatomes (Sensory Supply)

Investigations

- MRI is investigation of choice

Treatment

1. Rest and Anti-inflammatory Medications
   Continuous bed rest for 2 weeks will reduce the herniation in over 90%of cases.
2. If improvement is not complete epidural injection of corticosteroid and local anesthetic may help. **Back strengthening should be started only after pain has subsided.**
3. **Operative removal of disc** options are unilateral laminectomy/ Laminotomy or microscopic disc removal or endoscopic disc removal.

4. Chemonucleolysis dissolution of nucleus pulposus by percutaneous injection of proteolytic enzyme (chymopapain) is of theoretical significance.

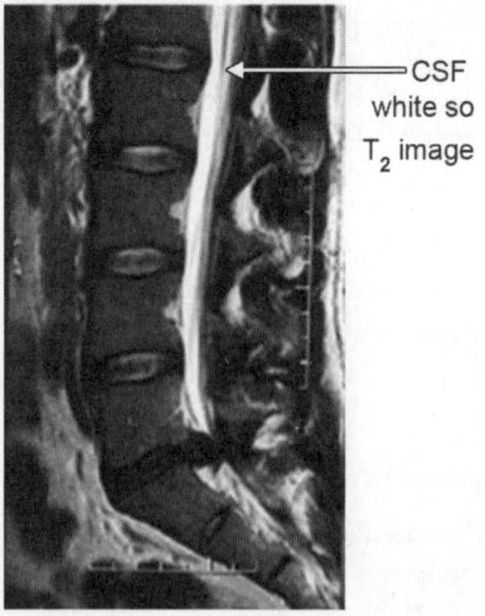

Fig. 13.2: MRI lumbosacral spine

Indications for Surgery

Absolute indications:

1. Bladder and bowel involvement
2. Increasing neurological deficit

Relative indications:

1. Failure of conservative treatment – Upto 6 weeks of trial is usually given
2. Recurrent sciatica : 1st attack 90% recover
   2nd attack 90% recover; 50% recurrent consider surgery.
   3rd attack 90% recover but all recurrent propose surgery
3. Significant neurological deficit with SLR reduction
4. Disc rupture in stenotic canal
5. Recurrent neurological deficit

SPONDYLOLISTHESIS AND SPONDYLOLYSIS

Spondylolisthesis is the slippage forward of one vertebrae upon another. It nearly always occurs between L5 and S1 (most common) or L4 and L5. Spondylolysis is characterized by presence of bony defect at pars interarticularis, which can result in spondylolisthesis.

DE QUERVAIN'S DISEASE

The abductor pollicis longus and extensor pollicis brevis tendons may become inflammed beneath the retinacular pulley at the radial styloid with in the first extensor compartment.

Pathognomic sign is Finkelstein's test. The examiner places patients' thumb across the palm in full flexion, and then holding the patient's hand firmly, turns the wrist sharply into adduction. In positive test this is acutely painful; repeating the movement with the thumb left free is relatively painless.

Differential diagnosis include scaphoid non-union, arthritis at the base of thumb and intersection syndrome.

Treatment

NSAIDS with splint if it fails than steroid injection into tendon sheath and if not relieved than treatment consists of splitting the thickened tendon sheath.

DUPUYTREN'S CONTRACTURE

This is nodular hypertrophy and contracture of superficial palmar fascia (palmar aponeurosis).

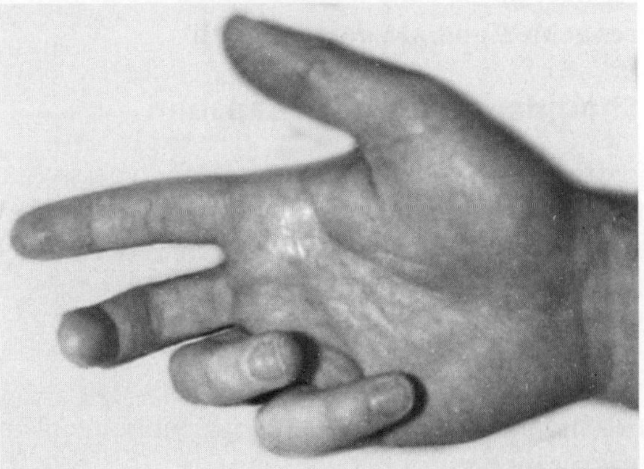

Fig. 13.3: Dupuytren's contracture ring finger and little finger involved

Epidemiology and Associations

Higher incidence in epileptics receiving phenytoin therapy, diabetics, alcoholic cirrhosis, AIDS, pulmonary tuberculosis.

Pathology

Proliferation of myofibroblast. Fibrous bands cause flexion deformity of MP and PIP joints and puckering of skin.

Ectopic deposits may occur in dorsum of PIP joint (Garrod's/ knuckle pads), sole of feet (Ledderhose's disease) and fibrosis of corpus cavernosum (Peyronie's disease).

Clinical Features

A middle aged man usually complains of nodular thickening of palm.

Flexion contracture most commonly occur at MP joint. >PIP joint> DIP joint .

Ring finger is involved followed by little finger

Table top test is positive

Treatment

Wait and watch

Collagenase has also been used

Subtotal fasciectomy is done its indications are flexion deformity >30 degrees at MCP and >15 degrees at PIP

Frozen Shoulder or Adhesive Capsulitis

The cardinal feature is stubborn lack of active and passive movement in all directions. i.e. global restriction of movements in all planes. Often the first motion to be affected is internal rotation followed by abduction. It is associated with diabetes mellitus.

Painful Arc Syndrome

It is anterior shoulder pain in 60 - 120° of glenohumeral abduction. Most common cause is.

Chronic supraspinatus tendinitis.

PULLED ELBOW/ NURSE MAID'S ELBOW

It is subluxation of radial head or more accurately subluxation of the annular (orbicular) ligament which slips up over the head of radius into the radiocapitellar joint.

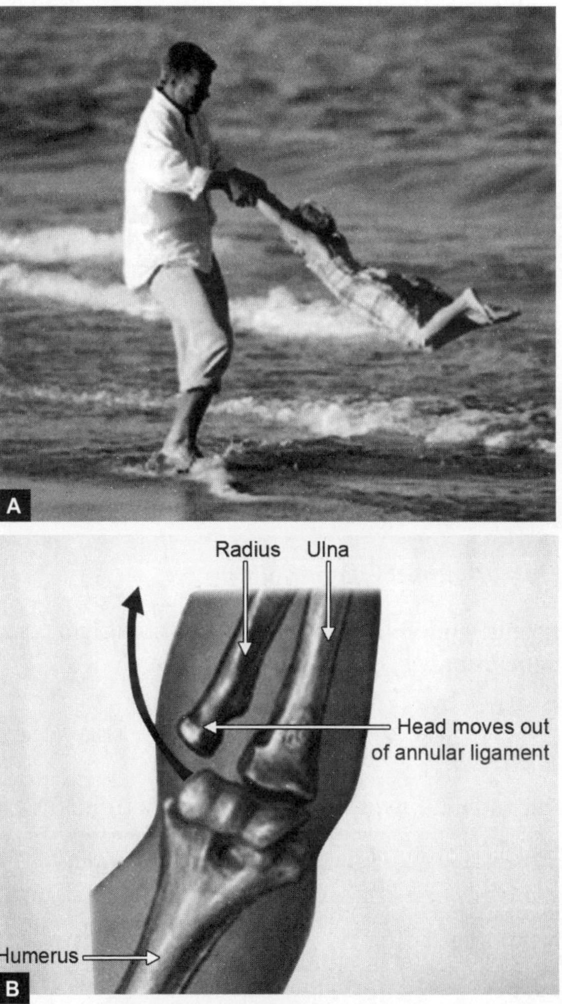

Figs. 13.4A and B: Pulled elbow

Mechanism of Injury

Traction to elbow

Clinical Features

- Maximum incidence in 1-4 years age group.
- The child holds the elbow in slight flexion with the forearm pronated.

X-rays are normal

Treatment

- Reduced by flexing the elbow to 90 degrees and rapidly and firmly rotating the forearm into full supination on outdoor basis without anaesthesia immobilization is not necessary.

Stenosing Flexor Tenosynovitis Trigger Finger

Due to stenosing tenosynovitis the flexor tendon may become trapped at the entrance to its fibrous digital sheath. The usual cause is thickening of fibrous tendon sheath or constriction of mouth of fibrous digital sheath. (mainly Al pulley) at the level of metacarpophalangeal joint.

Compound Palmar Ganglion

It is seen in Rheumatoid arthritis and Tuberculosis and causes hourglass swelling that goes beneath the flexor retinaculum.

Tennis Elbow/Lateral Epicondylitis

- It is chronic tendonitis of common extensor origin (esp. extensor carpi radialis brevis) on lateral epicondyle.

Cozen test is positive

Golfer's Elbow

Medial epicondylitis involving common flexor pronator origin.

Bursitis	Site
Student's Elbow/miners elbow	Olecranon bursitis
Housemaid's knee	Prepatellar bursitis
Clergyman's knee	Infrapatellar bursitis
Weaver's bottom	Ischial bursitis
Tailor's ankle	Lateral malleolus bursitis
Bunion	Medial side of great toe-1st metatarsal head bursitis
Bunionette	5th toe of foot-5th metatarsal head bursitis

QUESTIONS

1. The image shows presence of?

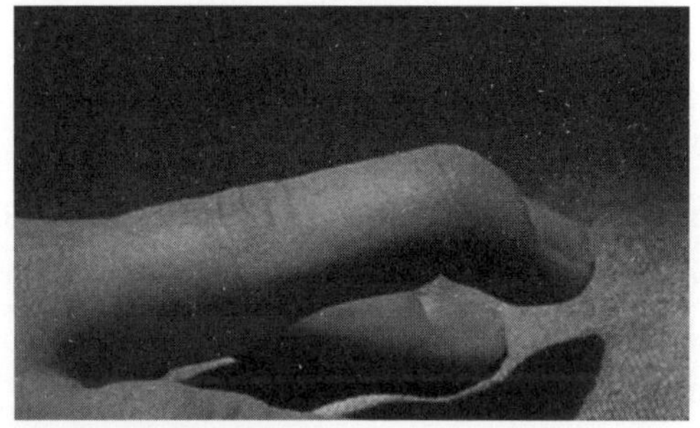

a. Swan neck deformity
b. Boutonnierre deformity
c. Mallet finger
d. Duputyren's contracture

Ans. is 'c' Mallet finger

2. Little finger of the hand corresponds to:

a. C6 dermatome
b. C7 dermatome
c. C8 dermatome
d. T1 dermatome

Ans. is 'c' C8 dermatome

3. Keller's operation is done for?

a. Hallux valgus
b. Hallux varus
c. Genu varus
d. CTEV

Ans. is 'a' Hallux valgus

4. Which ligament is involved in Pes-planus:

a. Spring ligament
b. Deep transverse ligament
c. Long & short plantar ligament
d. Deltoid ligament

Ans. is 'a' Spring ligament

5. Finkelstein test is done for:

a. Compound palmar ganglia

b. Carpal tunnel syndrome

c. De Quervain's tenosynovitis

d. Tennis elbow

Ans. is 'c' De Quervain's tenosynovitis

6. Dupuytren's contracture is associated with all EXCEPT:

a. Seen in cirrhosis

b. Involves the ring and little finger

c. Table top test is negative

d. Clostridial collagenase for resolution

Ans. is 'c' Table top test is negative

7. Pathognomonic sign of compound palmar ganglion is:

a. Swelling/edema of hand

b. Hourglass swelling above and below the flexor retinaculum

c. Rounded swelling above wrist

d. Reducible swelling

Ans. is 'b' Hourglass swelling above and below the flexor retinaculum

8. In the lumbar spine, 90% of the disc herniations occur at which of the following level:

a. L1-L2 b. L2-L3

c. L3-L4 d. L4-L5

Ans. is 'd' L4-L5

9. A tennis player presented with pain and tenderness at the lateral epicondyle of the humerus. These findings are c onsistent with the diagnosis of:

a. Tennis elbow

b. Golfer's elbow

c. Fibrositis

d. Dupuytren's contracture

Ans. is 'a' Tennis elbow

10. De Quervain's tenosynovitis is a stenosing tenosynovitis of the:

a. Tendo Achilles

b. Iliolumbar ligament

c. First extensor compartment of the wrist

d. Median nerve

Ans. is 'c' First extensor compartment of the wrist

11. Nursemaid's elbow is:

a. Elbow dislocation

b. Radial head subluxation (Pulled elbow)

c. Radial head fracture

d. Lateral epicondylitis

Ans. is 'b' Radial head subluxation (Pulled elbow)

12. Housemaid's knee is bursitis of which of the following:

a. Olecranon bursa b. Infrapatellar bursa

c. Prepatellar bursa d. Subacromial bursa

Ans. is 'c' Prepatellar bursa

13. Spondylolysis is more common in:

a. Intervertebral disc b. Anterior part

c. Pars interarticularis d. Annulus fibrosus

Ans. is 'c' Pars interarticularis

14. Clergyman's knee is:

a. Infrapatellar bursitis b. Semimembranosus bursitis

c. Prepatellar bursitis d. Suprapatellar bursitis

Ans. is 'a' Infrapatellar bursitis

15. A child is spinned around by his father by holding both hand's while doing this the child started crying and does not allow his father to touch the elbow. the diagnosis:

a. Annular ligament Tear b. Fracture olecranon process

c. Pulled elbow d. Radial head dislocation

Ans. is 'c' Pulled elbow

16. Dupuytrens contracture commonly affects:

(September 2005)

a. Little finger b. Ring finger

c. Middle finger d. Index finger

Ans. is 'b' is Ring finger

17. A 44-year-old man presented with acute onset of low backache radiating to the right lower limb. Examination revealed SLRT <400 on the right side, weakness of extensor hallucis longus on the right side, sensory loss in the first web space of the right foot and brisk knee jerk. Which of the following Is the most likely diagnosis:

(AIIMS May 04)

a. Prolapsed intervertebral disc L4-5

b. Spondylolysis L5-S1

c. Lumbar canal stenosis

d. Spondylolisthesis L4-5

Ans. is 'a' Prolapsed intervertebral disc L4-5

18. De Quervain's disease classically affects the:

a. Flexor pollicis longus and brevis

b. Extensor carpi radialis and extensor pollicis longus

c. Abductor pollicis longus and brevis

d. Extensor pollicis brevis and abductor pollicis longus

Ans. is 'd' Extensor pollicis brevis and abductor pollicis longus

19. In trigger finger the level of tendon sheath constriction is found at the level of:

a. Middle phalanx *(AIIMS May 05, AIIMS 96)*

b. Proximal interphalangeal joint

c. Proximal phalanx

d. Metacarpophalangeal joint

Ans. is 'd' Metacarpophalangeal joint

Chapter 14

Peripheral Nerve Injury

SEDDONS CLASSIFICATION

Neurapraxia: Tinels Sign Negative

- It is temporary physiological disruption of nerve impulse conduction. The loss of function is incomplete.
- Complete recovery takes place in 3-6 weeks and it comes back like lightening i.e. completely recovers in one go.
- No Wallerian degeneration takes place and Tinels sign is negative.
  - Crutch palsy - Pressure palsy (Radial nerve or part of brachial plexus injured)
  - Saturday night palsy - Pressure palsy
  - Tourniquet palsy - Pressure palsy
- Few Traumatic nerve injuries are neurapraxia

Axonotmesis: Tinels sign positive and progressive

- It is Axon breakdown, Tinels Sign is positive, Motor March is seen (Recovery of muscles takes place in the order of their Nerve Supply from proximal to distal direction).
- Recovery is usually not complete.
- Seen in closed fractures and dislocations

Neurotmesis: Tinels sign is positive and non-progressive

- Complete anatomic section of the nerve. Tinels Sign is positive and non-progressive.
- No recovery without surgical intervention. Even with intervention may not have complete recovery.
- Degeneration distal to injuries (Secondary or Wallerian degeneration)

- Degeneration in proximal segment (Primary or retrograde degeneration)
- At proximal end forms – Neuroma

Sunderland Classification in relation to seddons:

Type I	– Neurapraxia
Type II, III, IV	– Axonotmesis
Type V	– Neurotmesis

Autonomous Zone of Nerves: Exclusively Supplied by that Particular Nerve

- Median Nerve – Tip of index finger, Middle finger.
- Ulnar Nerve – Tip of little finger
- Radial Nerve – 1st web space on dorsum of hand
- Deep peroneal nerve – Dorsum of 1st web space on foot
- Tinel's Sign: (Records regeneration rate) by tapping on the nerve course from distal to proximal direction tingling is felt at the sprouting nerve ends and it disappears as myelinization takes place (Rate of Recovery of Nerve is 1mm/day) Tinels is positive and progressive in axonotmesis and sunderland 2 and 3.

EMG is the best test for nerve recovery

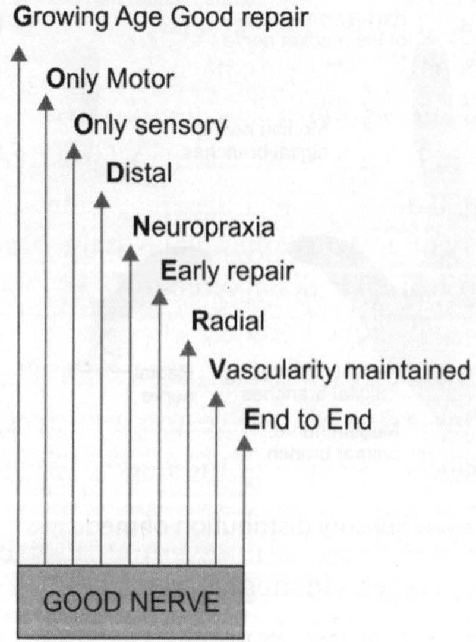

Rate of nerve regeneration – 1 mm/day (1 inch/month).

Nerve	Trauma	Effect
Axillary nerve	Dislocation of the shoulder (Anterior and Inferior)	Deltoid palsy
Radial nerve	Fracture shaft of the humerus (lower 1/3rd)	Wrist drop
Ulnar nerve	Fracture medial epicondyle humerus	Claw hand
Sciatic nerve	Posterior dislocation of the hip	Foot drop
Common peroneal nerve	Knee dislocation/Fracture of neck of the fibula	Foot drop
Posterior Interosseous Nerve	Monteggia fracture	Finger drop
Anterior interosseous nerve	Supra condylar fracture Humerus	Kiloh-Nevin sign
Median nerve	Supracondylar fracture of humerus	Pointing index

Median nerve palsy–Supplies nail bed of middle finger

1. Sensory supply

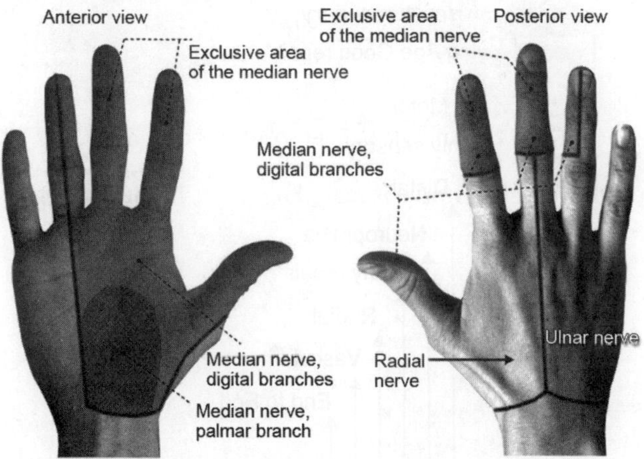

Fig. 14.1: Sensory distribution of median nerve

2. Partial claw hand is seen in median nerve palsy
3. Pointing index is seen due to paralysis of flexors of index and middle finger

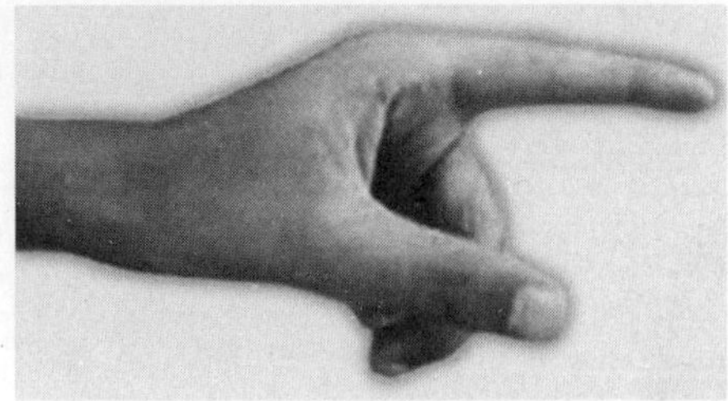

Fig. 14.2: Pointing index

4. Pen test is positive-due to paralysis of abductor pollicis brevis
5. Ape thumb deformity is seen
6. Opposition is lost with median nerve palsy
7. Splint used is Knuckle bender splint

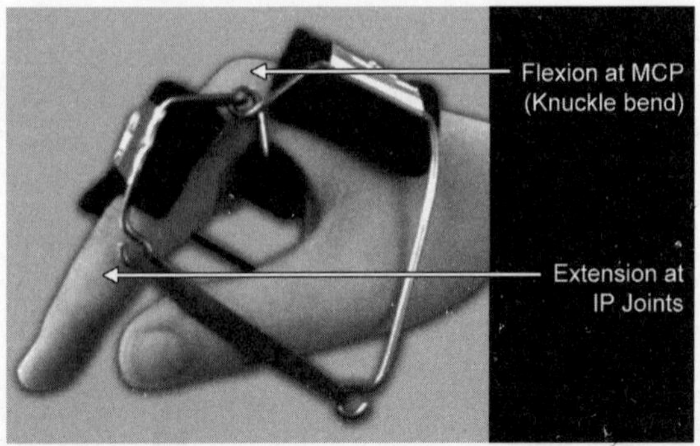

Fig. 14.3: Knuckle bender splint - for claw hand

Anterior interosseous nerve is tested by Kiloh-Nevin sign

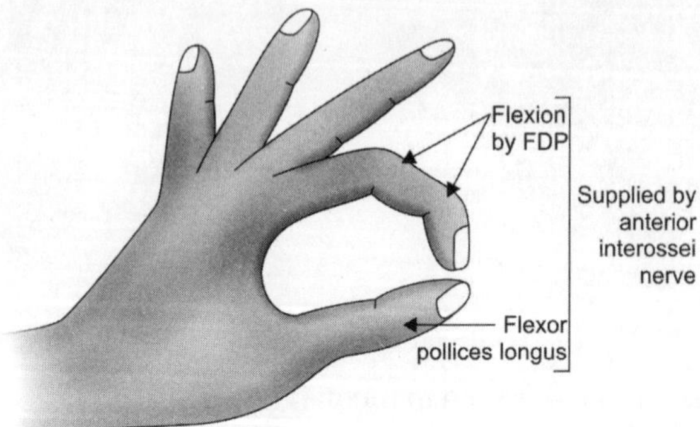

Fig. 14.4: AIN

Ulnar nerve palsy –Patient cannot adduct thumb.

1. Partial claw hand is seen in ulnar nerve palsy

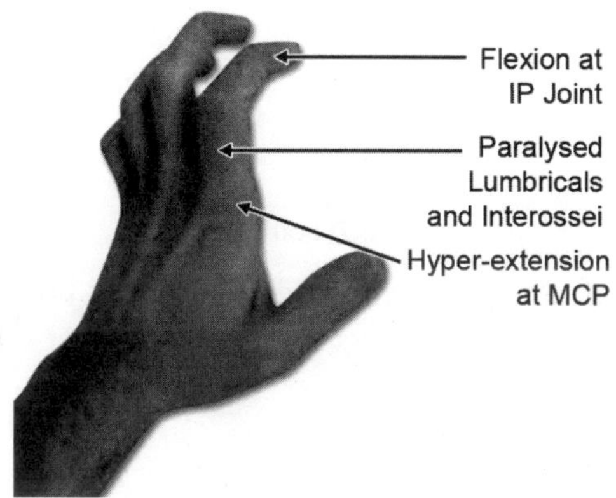

Fig. 14.5: Claw hand

2. Palmar interossei are paralysed hence adduction not possible hence holding card between the fingers is not possible.-Card test

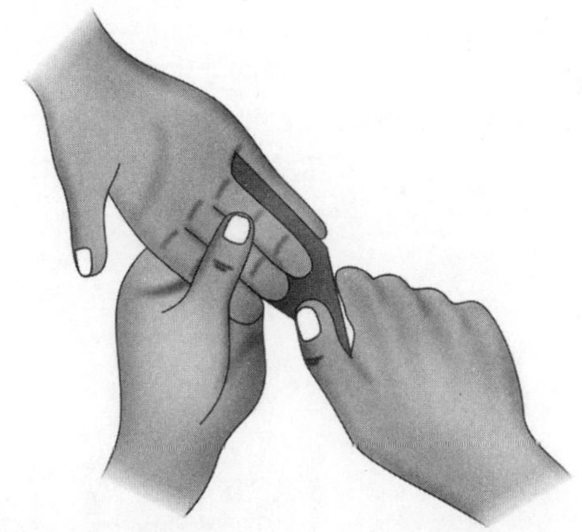

Fig. 14.6: Card test (Palmar interossei-adduction)

3. Igawa test is positive abduction of middle finger lost in ulnar nerve palsy causing paralysis of dorsal interossei
4. Book test–to-test adductor pollicis holding book between thumb and palm

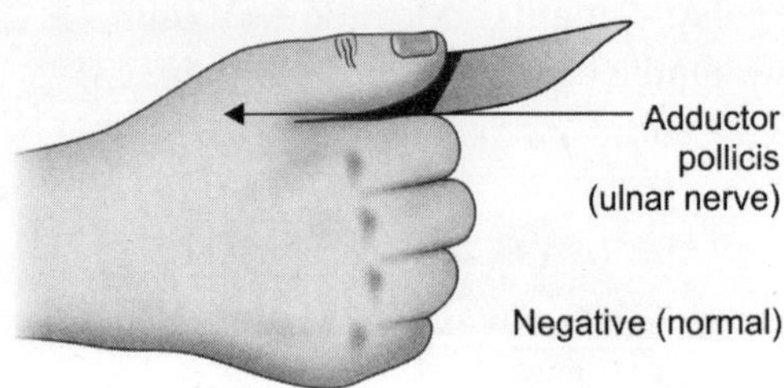

Fig. 14.7: Book test

5. Froment sign due to palsy of adductor pollicis book is held by flexion of index finger

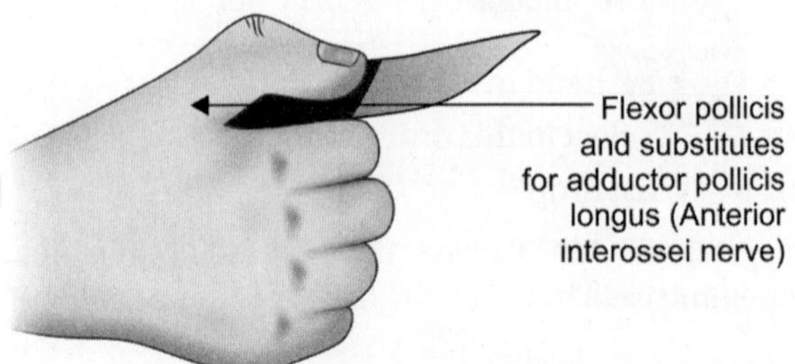

Fig. 14.8: Froment sign

6. Wartenberg sign-abducted little finger in ulnar nerve palsy

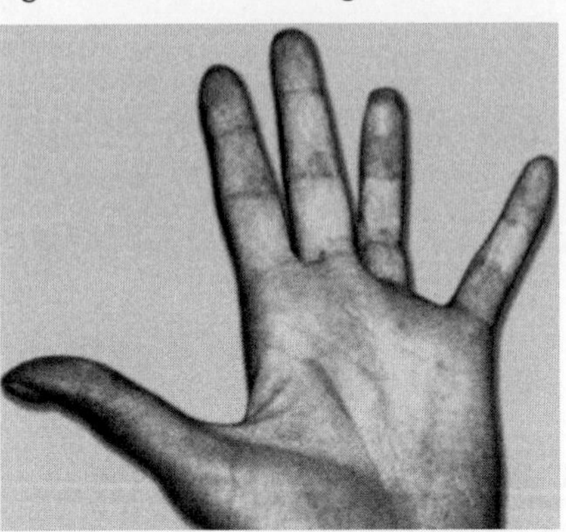

Fig. 14.9: Wartenberg sign

7. Splint used is Knuckle bender splint

Knuckle bender splint

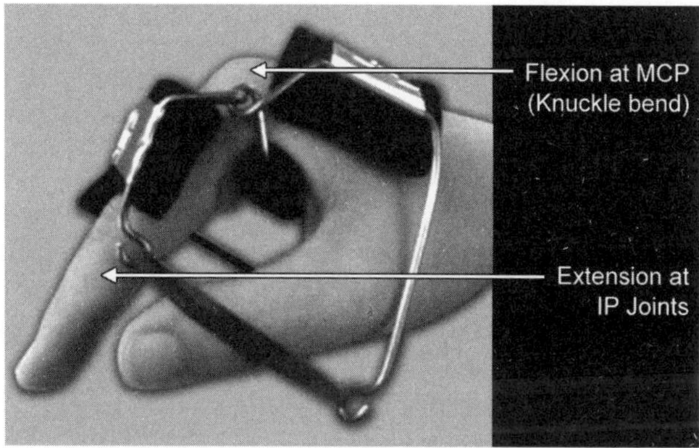

Fig. 14.10: Knuckle bender splint - for claw hand

Note Complete claw hand involves ulnar and median nerve.

Partial claw hand select in this order-Ulnar nerve >Median nerve.

Radial nerve – Wrist drop

Posterior interossei nerve palsy – Thumb drop or finger drop.

Cock up splint is used

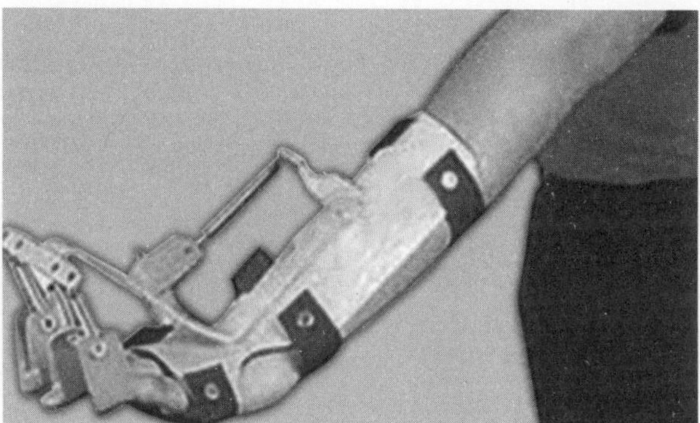

Fig. 14.11: Cock-up splint-for radial nerve

COMPRESSION NEUROPATHY

It is compression of a nerve in a closed space it is also called as entrapment neuropathy.

Carpal tunnel syndrome -compression of median nerve is the most common typed.

Most common cause of carpal tunnel syndrome is idiopathic. Other causes are Pregnancy, Hypothyroidism, Rheumatoid arthritis, Osteoarthritis, Acromegaly.

Sensory symptoms can often be reproduced by percussing over the median nerve (Tinel's sign) or by holding the wrist fully flexed for a minute or two (Phalen's test) or tourniquet test or Dunkans direct compression over median nerve (most reliable clinical test for median nerve).

Entrapment syndrome	Nerve involved
Carpal tunnel syndrome	Median nerve (at wrist) (Most Common)
Guyon's canal syndrome	Ulnar nerve (at wrist)
Cubital tunnel syndrome	Ulnar nerve (at elbow)
Meralgia paraesthetica	Lateral cutaneous nerve of thigh
Tarsal tunnel syndrome	Posterior tibial nerve (behind and below medial malleolus)

Femoral nerve is usually not involved in Nerve Entrapment Syndrome

NCV investigation of choice

Nerve palsy	Presentation
• Erb's palsy	Policeman tip deformity (Porter's tip deformity)
• Nerve of bell (Long thoracic nerve) palsy	Winging of scapula
• Median nerve palsy (Labours nerve)	Pointing index Bendiction test, Pen test (tests abductor pollicis brevis) Ochsner clasp test/Opposition of thumb lost /Ape thumb deformity
• Ulnar nerve palsy (Musician nerve)	Book test (Froment sign), Card test (PAD) – Palmar Interossei Igawa's test (DAB) – Dorsal interossei
• Radial nerve palsy	Wrist drop, (Finger drop and thumb dropSpecifically in posterior interosseous nerve (PIN) injury)
• Common peroneal nerve palsy (Lateral popliteal nerve palsy) or sciatic nerve palsy	Foot drop(complete)

Leprosy (Hansens disease)causes involvement of ulnar nerve at elbow and for foot drop most common tendon transfer is Tibialis posterior.

Hand knee gait is seen in poliomyelitis.

Brachial plexus most commonly -Erbs palsy (Policeman or waiters tip deformity) is palsy of upper trunk of brachial plexus. (C5, C6).

Movements lost in ERBS palsy are

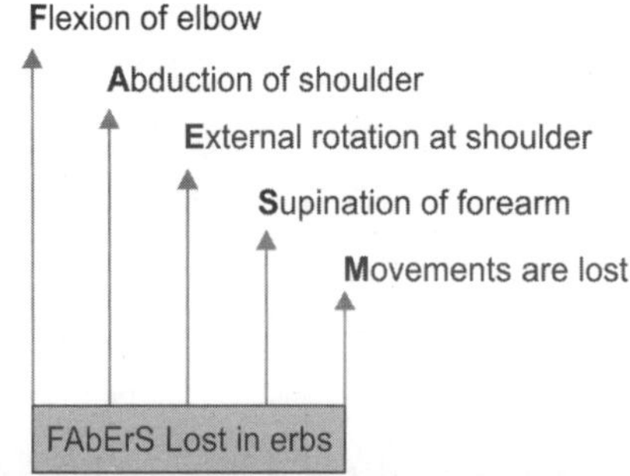

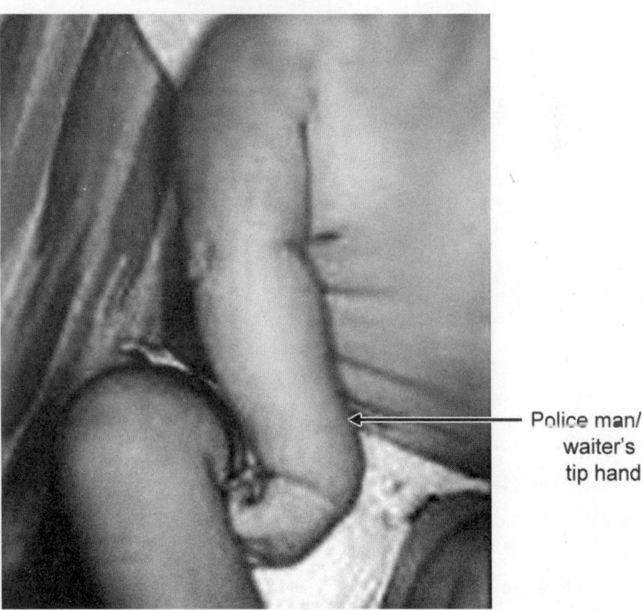

Fig. 14.12: Erbs palsy

Klumpbes paralysis is involvement of lower trunk of brachial plexus (C8,T1) causing claw hand.

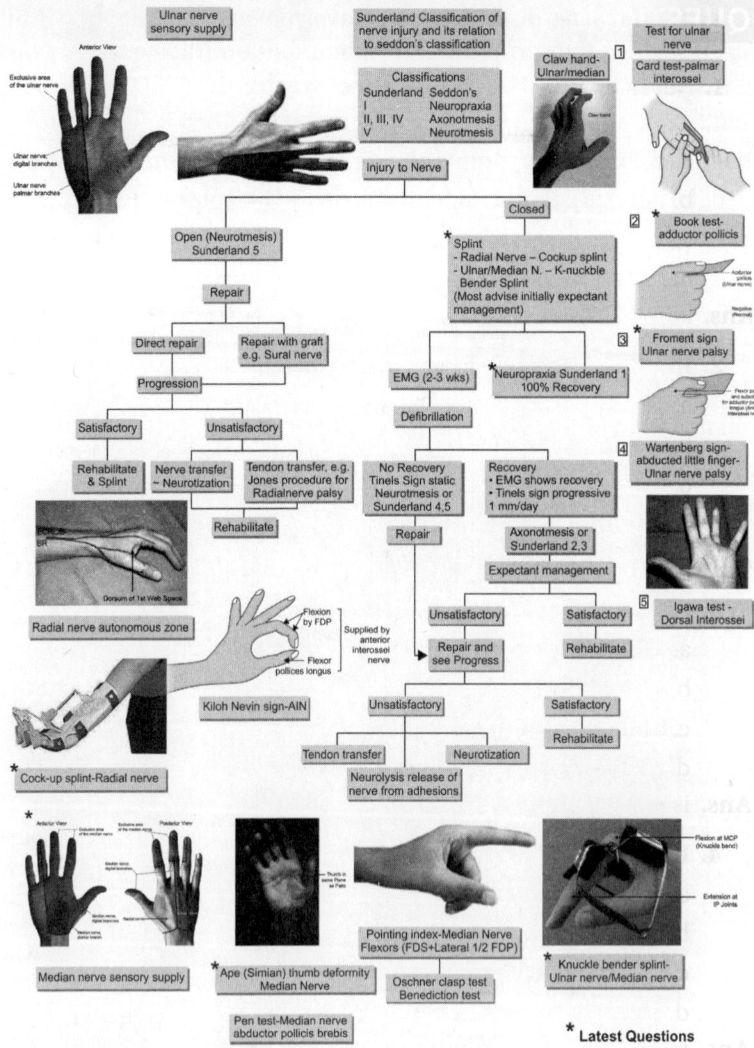
Ulnar nerve sensory supply
Anterior View
Exclusive area of the ulnar nerve
Ulnar nerve, digital branches
Ulnar nerve palmar branches
Sunderland Classification of nerve injury and its relation to seddon's classification
Classifications
Sunderland Seddon's
I Neuropraxia
II, III, IV Axonotmesis
V Neurotmesis
Injury to Nerve
Open (Neurotmesis) Sunderland 5
Repair
Direct repair
Repair with graft e.g. Sural nerve
Progression
Satisfactory
Unsatisfactory
Rehabilitate & Splint
Nerve transfer ~ Neurotization
Tendon transfer, e.g. Jones procedure for Radialnerve palsy
Rehabilitate
Closed
* Splint
- Radial Nerve – Cockup splint
- Ulnar/Median N. – K-nuckble Bender Splint
(Most advise initially expectant management)
EMG (2-3 wks)
* Neuropraxia Sunderland 1 100% Recovery
Defibrillation
No Recovery Tinels Sign static Neurotmesis or Sunderland 4,5
Repair
Recovery
• EMG shows recovery
• Tinels sign progressive 1 mm/day
Axonotmesis or Sunderland 2,3
Expectant management
Unsatisfactory
Satisfactory
Repair and see Progress
Rehabilitate
Unsatisfactory
Satisfactory
Rehabilitate
Tendon transfer
Neurotization
Neurolysis release of nerve from adhesions
Claw hand- Ulnar/median
Test for ulnar nerve
1 Card test-palmar interossei
2 * Book test- adductor pollicis
3 * Froment sign Ulnar nerve palsy
4 Wartenberg sign- abducted little finger- Ulnar nerve palsy
5 Igawa test - Dorsal Interossei
Dorsum of 1st Web Space
Radial nerve autonomous zone
Flexion by FDP
Flexor pollices longus
Supplied by anterior interossei nerve
Kiloh Nevin sign-AIN
* Cock-up splint-Radial nerve
* Anterior View
Posterior View
Median nerve sensory supply
* Ape (Simian) thumb deformity Median Nerve
Pen test-Median nerve abductor pollicis brebis
Pointing index-Median Nerve Flexors (FDS+Lateral 1/2 FDP)
Oschner clasp test Benediction test
Flexion at MCP (Knuckle bend)
Extension at IP Joints
* Knuckle bender splint- Ulnar nerve/Median nerve
* Latest Questions

QUESTIONS

1. **Nerve involved in carpal tunnel syndrome**

   (Recent Pattern Question 2016)

   a. Ulnar nerve
   b. Radial nerve
   c. Median nerve
   d. Medial nerve

Ans. is 'c' Median nerve

2. **Injury to cervical nerve C5, C6 causes:**
   a. Erb's paralysis
   b. Klumpke paralysis
   c. Horner syndrome
   d. Central cord syndrome

Ans. is 'a' Erb's paralysis

3. **Card test/book test is done for which nerve injury:**
   a. Radial nerve
   b. Ulnar nerve
   c. Median nerve
   d. Tibial nerve

Ans. is 'b' Ulnar nerve

4. **Ulnar nerve paralysis causes:**
   a. Ape thumb deformity
   b. Wrist drop
   c. Claw finger deformity
   d. Meralgia perasthetica

Ans. is 'c' Claw finger deformity

5. **Neurapraxia is a condition characterized by:**
   a. Division of nerve sheath
   b. Division of axons
   c. Division of nerve fibres
   d. Physiological block

Ans. is 'd' Physiological block

6. Pain due to postamputation neuroma is best treated by:

a. Infrared therapy
b. Interference therapy
c. Ultrasound therapy
d. Stump bandaging

Ans. is 'b' Interference therapy

7. The picture given below shows a hand following a nerve injury. Identify the nerve:

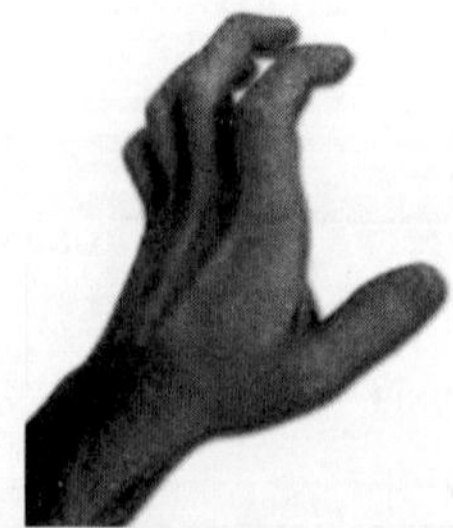

a. Axillary nerve
b. Ulnar nerve
c. Radial nerve
d. Musculocutaneous nerve

Ans. is 'b' Ulnar nerve

8. Nerve involved in foot drop is?

a. Deep peroneal
b. Common peroneal
c. Anterior tibial
d. Posterior tibial

Ans. is 'b' Common peroneal

9. Axillary nerve damage is caused by damage to?

a. Shaft of humerus
b. Surgical neck humerus
c. Medial epicondyle
d. Lateral epicondyle

Ans. is 'b' Surgical neck humerus

10. Phalen test is done for?

a. De Quervain's tenosynovitis
b. Carpal tunnel syndrome
c. Rotator cuff injury
d. Tennis elbow

Ans. is 'b' Carpal tunnel syndrome

11. Most common cause of Sciatic nerve damage:

a. Degenerative
b. Iatrogenic
c. Traumatic
d. Vascular

Ans. is 'c' Traumatic

12. Which nerve injured in fracture of fibula:

a. Posterior tibial nerve
b. Anterior tibial nerve
c. Common peroneal nerve
d. Deep peroneal nerve

Ans. is 'c' Common peroneal nerve

13. Motor march is seen in:

a. Neurapraxia
b. Axonotmesis
c. Neurotmesis
d. None of these

Ans. is 'b' Axonotmesis

14. Which of the following DOESN'T indicate ulnar nerve injury:

a. Clawing of medial 2 digits
b. Froment sign is present
c. Abductor pollicis longus palsy
d. Loss of sensory supply of medial little finger and medial half of ring finger

Ans. is 'c' Abductor pollicis longus palsy

15. A women aged 30 years pregnant after trauma feeling tingling pain and numbness at the tip of thumb, index finger and middle finger, on examination doctor pressed between the wrist joint for 30 seconds and the patients develops more pain at the tips of the middle, index finger and thumb what is the diagnosis:

a. Carpal tunnel syndrome
b. Cubital tunnel syndrome
c. Meralgia Paresthetica
d. Tarsal tunnel syndrome

Ans. is 'a' Carpal tunnel syndrome

16. What is Neurapraxia:

a. Complete division of nerve
b. Loss of conduction due to axonal interruption
c. Irreversible injury
d. Reversible physiological nerve conduction block

Ans. is 'd' Reversible physiological nerve conduction block

17. Neurapraxia is defined as: *(March 2012)*

a. Anatomically normal but physiological interruption of nerve conduction
b. Nerve intact with broken axons
c. Axons as well as nerve broken
d. None of the above

Ans. is 'a' Anatomically normal but physiological interruption of nerve conduction

18. Tinel sign indicates:

a. Nerve degeneration
b. Nerve regeneration
c. Both
d. None

Ans. is 'b' Nerve regeneration

19. After repair of an injured peripherals nerve the estimated rate of functional recovery per month is:

a. ½ inch
b. 1 inch
c. 1.5 inch
d. 2 inch

Ans. is 'b' 1 inch

20. Nerve supply of nail bed of middle finger:

a. Radial nerve *(March 2013)*
b. Ulnar nerve
c. Median nerve
d. Axillary nerve

Ans. is 'c' Median nerve

21. Pen test & Benediction sign is seen in:

a. Radial nerve involvement

b. Median nerve involvement

c. Ulnar nerve involvement

d. Axillary nerve involvement

Ans. is 'b' Median nerve involvement

22. Pointing index is because of :

a. Median nerve injury

b. Radial nerve injury

c. 1st metacarpal fracture

d. Ulnar nerve injury

Ans. is 'a' Median nerve injury

23. Froment's sign is a feature of:

a. Radial nerve palsy

b. Ulnar nerve palsy

c. Median nerve palsy

d. Tibial nerve palsy

Ans. is 'b' Ulnar nerve palsy

24. In the forearm the ulnar nerve supplies the:

a. Flexor pollicis longus

b. Pronator teres

c. Flexor profundus medial part

d. Flexor sublimis

Ans. is 'c' Flexor profundus medial part

25. Inability to adduct the thumb is due to the injury of:

a. Median nerve

b. Ulnar nerve

c. Radial nerve

d. Musculocutaneous nerve

Ans. is 'b' Ulnar nerve

26. Knuckle bender splint is used for:

a. Ulnar nerve palsy

b. Radial nerve palsy

c. Median nerve palsy

d. Axillary nerve palsy

Ans. is 'a' Ulnar nerve palsy

27. Total claw hand is seen in the paralysis of:

a. Ulnar and median nerveb. Ulnar nerve

c. Median nerve

d. Radial nerve

Ans.. is 'a' Ulnar and median nerve

28. Partial claw hand is caused by lesion involving the:

a. Radial nerve b. Ulnar nerve

c. Median nerve d. Anterior interosseous nerve

Ans. is 'b' Ulnar nerve

29. A "true claw-hand" of severe type results from:

a. A lesion of the ulnar nerve at the elbow

b. A lesion of the median nerve at the elbow

c. A combined lesion of median and ulnar nerves at the elbow

d. A combined lesion of ulnar and radial nerves at the elbow

Ans. is 'c' A combined lesion of median and ulnar nerves at the elbow

30. Fractures of fibular neck may involve: *(March 2012)*

a. Tibial nerve b. Sciatic nerve

c. Common peroneal nerve

d. Sural nerve

Ans. is 'c' Common peroneal nerve

31. Foot drop occurs due to the involvement of:

a. Sciatic nerve

b. Direct injury to the dorsiflexors

c. Common peroneal nerve palsy

d. All of the above

Ans. is 'd' All of the above

32. Foot drop is due to all except:

a. Common peroneal nerve involvement.

b. Deep peroneals nerve involvement.

c. Sciatic nerve involvement

d. Posterior tibial nerve involvement

Ans. is 'd' Posterior tibial nerve involvement

33. Cockup splint is used in paralysis of:

a. Ulnar nerve b. Radial nerve

c. Median nerve d. Sciatic nerve

Ans. is 'b' Radial nerve

34. Which of the following serve as donors for nerve grafting procedures:

a. Spinal accessory nerve b. Superior mental nerve

c. Sural nerve d. Anterior interosseous nerve

Ans. is 'c' Sural nerve

35. Carpal tunnel syndrome is due to involvement of which nerve:

a. Radial nerve b. Median nerve

c. Ulnar nerve d. Axillary nerve

Ans. is 'b' Median nerve

36. Most common cause of Carpal tunnel syndrome is:

a. Renals failure b. Pregnancy

c. Arthritis d. Gont

e. Idiopathic

Ans. is 'e' Idiopathic

37. Carpal tunnel is associated with all of the following except:

a. Hyperparathyroidism b. Rheumatoid arthritis

c. Wrist osteoarthritis d. Acromegaly

Ans. is 'a' Hyperparathyroidism

38. Nerve compressed in Guyon's canal is: *(September 2003)*

a. Median and ulnar b. Median

c. Ulnar d. Radial

Ans. is 'c' Ulnar

39. Tarsal tunnel syndrome is:

a. Compression neuropathy of the posterior tibial nerve

b. Comminuted fractures of multiple tarsales with compartment syndrome.

c. Compression neuropathy of the femoral nerve

d. Sub astragalar arthritis

Ans. is 'a' Compression neuropathy of the posterior tibial nerve

40. Cubital tunnel syndrome involves: *(March 2013 (c, f))*

a. Radial nerve
b. Ulnar nerve
c. Median nerve
d. Axillary nerve

Ans. is 'b' Ulnar nerve

41. Hand-knee gait is seen in patients of: *(March 2013 (b, e))*

a. Leprosy
b. TB
c. Polio
d. Common peroneal nerve palsy

Ans. is 'c' Polio

42. Posterior dislocation of Hip can damage which nerve: *(NEET/DNB Pattern)*

a. Superior gluteal
b. Sciatic
c. Inferior gluteal
d. Femoral

Ans. is 'b' Sciatic.

43. The most popular tendon transfer for foot drop in leprosy:

a. Tibialis anterior laterally
b. Peromens longus to the dorsum
c. Tibialis posterior to the dorsum
d. Extensor hallucis longus to the metatarsals neck

Ans. is 'c' Tibialis posterior to the dorsum

44. In Erb's palsy, the classical "Policeman's tip" hand positions results due to the combination of all of the following deformities except:

a. Adduction at the shoulder
b. Extension at the elbow
c. External rotation of the arm
d. Pronation of the forearm

Ans. is 'c' External rotation of the arm

45. Tinel sign is used for: *(NEET/DNB Pattern)*

a. To assess the severity of damage of nerve
b. To classify the type of nerve injury
c. To locate the site of nerve injury
d. To assess the recovery

Ans. is 'd' To assess the recovery

46. Median nerve Injury at the wrist causes: *(PGI 98)*

a. Claw hand
b. Loss of apposition of thumb
c. Policeman's tip deformity
d. Saturday night palsy

Ans. is 'b' Loss of apposition of thumb

47. Compression of a nerve within the carpal tunnel products inability to: *(AIIMS May 05)*

a. Abduct the thumb
b. Adduct the thumb
c. Flex the distal phalanx of the thumb
d. Oppose the thumb

Ans. is 'd' Oppose the thumb

48. Pointing index sign is seen in — nerve palsy: *(AIIMS 97)*

a. Ulnar
b. Radial
c. Median
d. Axillazy

Ans.. is 'c' Median

49. Ape thumb deformity is seen In Involvement of: *(AI 2K, NEET/DNB Pattern)*

a. Median nerve
b. Ulnar nerve
c. Radial nerve
d. Axillary nerve

Ans. is 'a' Median nerve

50. A boy presents with complaints of hypoaesthesia and wasting of thenar eminence. The nerve most likely to be damaged in this patient: *(AIIMS 02)*

a. Musculocutaneous nerve
b. Median nerve
c. Ulnar nerve
d. Radial nerve

Ans. is 'b' Median nerve

51. Nerve damaged due to lunate dislocation (in carpal tunnel): *(PGI 2000)*

a. Median & ulnar
b. Median
c. Ulnar
d. Radial

Ans. is 'b' Median

52. Ulnar nerve injury at wrist involves following except: *(PGI 98)*

a. Palmar interossei
b. Opponens pollicis
c. Dorsal interossei
d. Adductor pollicis

Ans. is 'b' Opponens pollicis

53. Froment's sign is characteristically seen in: *(AIIMS June 97, May 93, DPG 94, NEET/ DNB Pattern)*

a. Ulnar nerve injury
b. Median nerve injury
c. Radial nerve injury
d. Intercostobrachial nerve injury

Ans. is 'b' Median nerve injury

54. Claw hand is caused by lesion of: *(AI 07)*

a. Ulnar nerve b. Median nerve
c. Axillary nerve d. Radial nerve

Ans. is 'a' Ulnar nerve

55. A 30-year-old male underwent excision of the right radial head. Following surgery the patient developed inability to extend the fingers and thumb of the right hand. He did not have any sensory deficit. Which one of the following is the most likely cause? *(AIIMS May 04)*

a. Injury to Posterior interosseus nerve
b. latrogenic injury to common extensor origin
c. Injury to anterior interosseus nerve
d. High radial nerve palsy

Ans. is 'a' Injury to Posterior interosseus nerve

56. A person is not able to extend his metacarpo-phalangeal joint. This is due to injury to which nerve: *(AIIMS June 00)*

a. Ulnar nerve
b. Radial nerve injury
c. Median nerve injury
d. Post. Interosseous nerve injury

Ans. is 'b' Radial nerve injury

57. A 19-year-old boy fell from the motorbike on his shoulder. The doctor diagnosed him a case of Erbs paralysis. The following signs and symptoms will be observed except: *(AIIMS 02)*

a. Loss of abduction at shoulder joint
b. Loss of lateral rotation
c. Loss of pronation at radioulnar joint
d. Loss of flexion at elbow joint

Ans. is 'c' Loss of pronation at radioulnar joint

58. A pole vaulter had a fall during pole vaulting and had paralysis of the arm. Which of the following investigations gives the best recovery prognosis: *(AIIMS Nov 03)*

a. Electromyography
b. Muscle biopsy
c. Strength Duration Curve
d. Creatine phosphokinase levels

Ans. is 'a' Electromyography

59. Most common cause of neurological deficit in upper limb is:

a. Polio *(AIIMS Nov 93)*
b. Erb's palsy
c. C-C2 dislocation
d. Fracture dislocation of cervical spine

Ans. is 'b' Erb's palsy

60. All the following nerves are involved in entrapment neuropathy except: *(AI 09)*

a. Femoral nerve
b. Median nerve
c. Ulnar nerve
d. Lateral cutaneous nerve of thigh

Ans. is 'a' Femoral nerve

61. Meralgia paresthetica is due to involvement of: *(AIIMS Dec 06, May 10)*

a. Medial cutaneous nerve of thigh
b. Lateral cutaneous nerve of thigh
c. Sural nerve
d. Femoral nerve

Ans. is 'b' Lateral cutaneous nerve of thigh

62. Carpal tunnel syndrome is due to compression of: *(AI 02)*

a. Radial nerve
b. Ulnar nerve
c. Palmer branch of the Ulnar nerve
d. Median nerve

Ans. is 'd' Median nerve

63. Carpal tunnel syndrome all are present except: *(NEET/DNB Pattern)*

a. Ulnar nerve dysfunction
b. Tinel sign
c. C) Phalens sign
d. Pain & paraesthesia of wrist

Ans. is 'a' Ulnar nerve dysfunction

64. A 56-years old female presents with nocturnal pain in the right thumb, index and middle fingers for the past 3 months. All of the provocative tests can be performed except: *(AIIMS Nov 11)*

a. Finkelstein's test
b. Tinel sign
c. Phalen's test
d. Tourniquet test

Ans. is 'a' Finkelstein's test

65. Trauma to neck of humerus, nerve damaged: *(NEET/DNB Pattern)*

a. Radial
b. b)Ulnar
c. Median
d. Axillary

Ans. is 'd' Axillary

Chapter 15

Joint Disorders

Synovial Fluid

Synovial Fluid: It is an ultradialysate of blood plasma transudated from synovial capillaries to which hyaluronic acid protein complex (mucin) has been added by synovial B cells.

Osteoarthritis

Osteoarthritis characteristically involves distal interphalangeal joint (Heberden's node), proximal interphalangeal joint (Bouchard's node) 1 carpometacarpal joint (base of thumb) of hand **with sparing of metacarpophalangeal joint and wrist joint.**

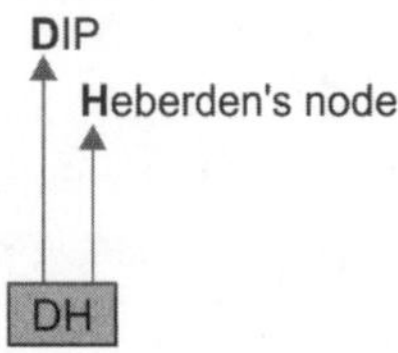

Due to decreased loading of painful extremity quadriceps weakness is common in patients of osteoarthritis of knee. Most importantly Vastus medialis is affected.

(AIIMS Nov 2011, AIPG 2007, AIIMS May 2007, AIPG 2011)

Classification system and stage wise management for OA knee

- Initial treatment is always conservative
- Clinical picture is more significant than radiology or X-ray changes
- If activities of daily living are affected surgery is advised
- Surgery for young is High Tibial Osteotomy
- Surgery for elderly (>60 years) is Total Knee Replacement

Rheumatoid Arthritis

Classification Criteria for Rheumatoid Arthritis - 2010		Score
Joint involvement	1 large joint (shoulder, elbow, hip, knee, ankle)	0
	2–10 large joints	1
	1–3 small joints (MCP, PIP, Thumb IP, MTP, wrists)	2
	4–10 small joints	3
	>10 joints (at least 1 small joint)	5
Serology	Negative RF and negative anti-CCP antibodies	0
	Low-positive RF or low-positive anti-CCP antibodies (3 times ULN)	2
	High-positive RF or high-positive anti-CCP antibodies (>3 times ULN)	3
Acute-phase reactants	Normal CRP and normal ESR	0
	Abnormal CRP or abnormal ESR	1
Duration of symptoms	<6 weeks	0
	>6 weeks	1

Total Score 10

Score $\geq$ 6 indicates – R.A

RF – Rheumatoid factor

anti-CCP antibodies - anti - Citrullinated Cyclic phosphate antibodies. It is positive in upto 98% of patient. 2% of general population has anti CCP positive.

The 1987 Revised Criteria for Diagnosis of RA

1. Guidelines for classification 4 of 7 criterion are required to classify a patient as having RA Patients with 2 or more criteria are not excluded.
2. Criteria (a - d must be present for at least 6 weeks and b- e must be observed by physician)
   a. Morning stiffness, in and around joint lasting 1 hour before maximal improvement.

b. Arthritis of 3 or more joint areas, observed by a physician simultaneously, have soft tissue swelling or joint effusion, not just bony over growth. The 14 possible joint areas involved are right or left proximal interphalangeal (PIP), metacarpophalangeal (MCP), wrist, elbow, knee, ankle and metatarsophalangeal joints (MTP).
c. Arthritis of hand joints e.g. wrist, MP or PIP joints.
d. Symmetrical arthritis i.e. simultaneous involvement of same joint area on both sides of body.
e. Rheumatoid nodules (Pathognomonic): subcutaneous nodules over bony prominences, extensor surfaces or juxta articular region.
f. Serum rheumatoid factor.
g. Radiological changes: bony erosion or unequivocal bony decalcification, periarticular osteoporosis and narrowing of articular (joint) space.

Distal Inter Phalangeal Joint is Usually Spared

Significance of Rheumatoid Factor (RF)

If present in high titre, to designates patients at risk for severe systemic disease.

'Swan - neck deformity' i.e. hyperextension of PIP joints with compensatory flexion of the distal interphalangeal joints

Boutonniere deformity i.e. flexion contracture of PIP joints and extension of DIP joints.

Poor Prognostic Factors of RA

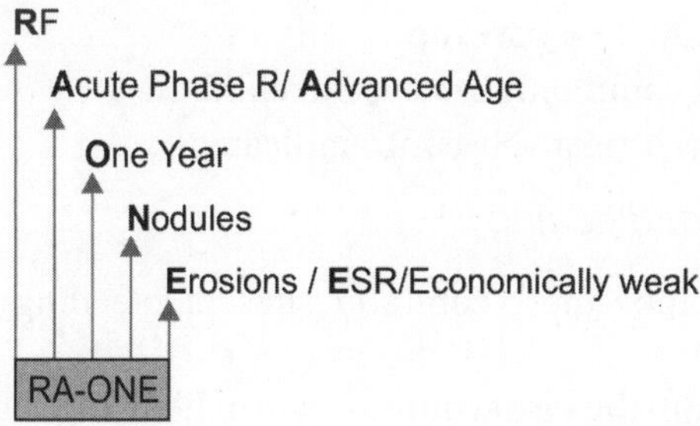

Pattern of Joint Involvement

	Osteoarthritis	Rheumatoid Arthritis	Psoriatic Arthritis
Involved	PIP, DIP and 1' CMC (corpometacarpal) joints	PIP, MCP, wrist	DIP, PIP and any joint
Spared	MCP (metacarpo phalangeal) and wrist	DIP joint	Sparing of any joint

Ankylosing Spondylitis (AS)/ Marie- Strumpell or Bechterew's Disease

Diagnostic Criteria – Modified New York Criterion

- Essential criteria is definite radiographic sacroiliitis
- Supporting criteria: one of these three
  - Inflammatory back pain
  - Limited chest expansion (<5 cm at 4th ICS) not a reliable criterion in elderly because of pulmonary disorders
  - Limited lumbar spine motion in both sagittal and frontal plane (Schober test /Modified Schober test).

Never diagnose Ankylosing spondylitis without sacroilitis

HLA B27 is associated with Ankylosing Spondylitis

Bamboo spine in seen in Ankylosing spondylitis

Hemophilic Arthropathy

Joint Bleeding

- Weight bearing joints are most commonly involved, with the frequency of involvement in decreasing order, knee>elbow> shoulder> ankle> wrist> hip
- Ankle most commonly involved in children
- Arthroscopy is relatively contraindicated.

Intramuscular Bleeding

- In lower limbs most common sites of bleeding is iliopsoas> quadriceps
- In upper limb the most common site of bleeding is deltoid

- Most hemophilic pseudotumors are caused by subperiosteal hemorrhage and the most common location is in thigh (50%). Next in frequency are abdomen, pelvis, and tibia.

Neuropathic Joint Disease/Charcot's Joint

It is progressive destructive arthritis arising from loss of pain sensation and proprioception (position sense). Diabetes mellitus (most common) cause. Joints involved are **Midtarsal (most common)** > tarsometatarsal metatarsophalangeal and ankle joint.

Disease	Joint Involvement
Diabetes	Midtarsal (most common)> tarsometatarsal, metatarsophalangeal and ankle joint> knee and spine
Tabes dorsalis	Knee(most common), hip, ankle and lumbar spine
Leprosy	Hand and foot joints
Syringomyelia	Shoulder (glenohumeral), elbow, wrist and cervical spine
Myelomeningocele	Ankle and foot
Congenital insensitivity to pain	Ankle and foot
Chronic Alcoholism	Foot
Amyloidosis	Peroneal Muscle atrophy (Charcot Marie tooth disease)

- The appearance suggest that movements would be agonizing and yet it is often painless.
- The paradox is diagnostic the amount of pain experienced is less than would be anticipated based on degree of joint involvement.
- Usual treatment is bracing or arthrodesis, total ankle Replacement is contraindicated.

Congenital Syphilis

Clutton's joint is painless, symmetrical, sterile effusion mostly involving knee in 8-16 years of age. Spontaneous remission is usual in several weeks.

- Non erosive arthritis : SLE
- Non deforming arthritis : Behcets

Disease	Area involved
• Septic	Knee
• Syphilitic arthritis*	Knee
• Gonococcal arthritis*	Knee
• Gout*	MP joint of big toe
• Pseudogout*	Knee
• Rheumatoid arthritis	Metacarpophalangeal joint
• Ankylosing spondylitis*	Sacroiliac joint
• Diabetic charcot joint*	Foot joint (tarsals)
• Senile osteoporosis*	Vertebra
• Pagets disease*	Pelvic bones > Femur > Skull > Tibia
• Osteochondritis dissecans*	Knee
• Actinomycosis*	Mandible
• Haemophilic arthritis*	Knee
• Disc prolapse*	Between L4 and L5
• Acute Osteomyelitis*	Lower end of femur (Metaphysis)
• Brodies Abscess*	Upper end of Tibia
• Pseudogout	

Feature	Gout (Protein Alcohol Intake)	Pseudogout (Hpothyroidism associated)
Synovial fluid Analysis	Uric acid crystal Needle or rod shaped crystal, Negatively birefringent crystals	Calcium pyrophosphate crystal, Rhomboid shaped crystal, Postive birefringent crystals
Associated with	ACTH, glucocorticoid withdrawal, hypouricemic therapy. Hperuricaemia. "Alcohol and Protein Intake"	Four 'H' S i.e. hyperparathyroidism, hemochromatosis, hypophophatasia, hypomagnesemia are associated. Most common association is Hypothyroidism Chondrocalcinosis i.e. appearance of calcific material articular cartilage and menisci is seen.
Clinicalpresentation	Intense pain	Moderate pain
Involved Joint	Smaller joints (most commonly metatarsophalangeal joint of big toe)	Larger joints most commonly, knee

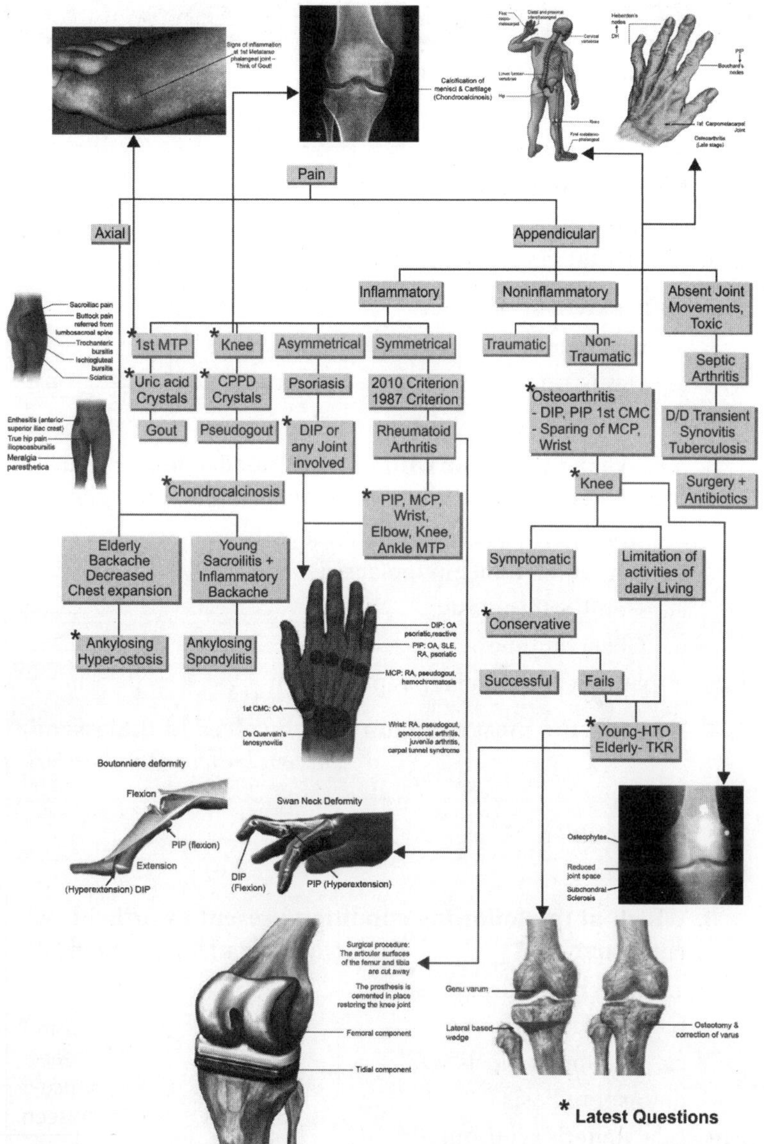
Signs of inflammation at 1st Metatarso phalangeal joint – Think of Gout!
Calcification of menisci & Cartilage (Chondrocalcinosis)
Heberden's nodes
Bouchard's nodes
1st Carpometacarpal Joint
Osteoarthritis (Late stage)
Pain
Axial
Appendicular
Inflammatory
Noninflammatory
Absent Joint Movements, Toxic
Sacroiliac pain
Buttock pain referred from lumbosacral spine
Trochanteric bursitis
Ischiogluteal bursitis
Sciatica
Enthesitis (anterior superior iliac crest)
True hip pain iliopsoasbursitis
Meralgia paresthetica
*1st MTP
*Knee
Asymmetrical
Symmetrical
Traumatic
Non-Traumatic
Septic Arthritis
*Uric acid Crystals
*CPPD Crystals
Psoriasis
2010 Criterion 1987 Criterion
*Osteoarthritis - DIP, PIP 1st CMC - Sparing of MCP, Wrist
D/D Transient Synovitis Tuberculosis
Gout
Pseudogout
*DIP or any Joint involved
Rheumatoid Arthritis
*Chondrocalcinosis
*Knee
Surgery + Antibiotics
*PIP, MCP, Wrist, Elbow, Knee, Ankle MTP
Elderly Backache Decreased Chest expansion
Young Sacroilitis + Inflammatory Backache
Symptomatic
Limitation of activities of daily Living
*Ankylosing Hyper-ostosis
Ankylosing Spondylitis
*Conservative
DIP: OA psoriatic,reactive
PIP: OA, SLE, RA, psoriatic
MCP: RA, pseudogout, hemochromatosis
1st CMC: OA
De Quervain's tenosynovitis
Wrist: RA, pseudogout, gonococcal arthritis, juvenile arthritis, carpal tunnel syndrome
Successful
Fails
*Young-HTO Elderly- TKR
Boutonniere deformity
Flexion
PIP (flexion)
Extension
(Hyperextension) DIP
Swan Neck Deformity
DIP (Flexion)
PIP (Hyperextension)
Osteophytes
Reduced joint space
Subchondral Sclerosis
Surgical procedure: The articular surfaces of the femur and tibia are cut away
The prosthesis is cemented in place restoring the knee joint
Femoral component
Tidial component
Genu varum
Lateral based wedge
Osteotomy & correction of varus
* Latest Questions

QUESTIONS

1. **Heberden's arthropathy affects:**
   a. Lumber spine *(Recent Pattern Question 2018)*
   b. Sacroiliac joint
   c. Distal interphalangeal joint
   d. Knee joint

Ans. is 'c' Distal interphalangeal joint

2. **Main extensor of knee:**
   a. Gastrocnemius b. Quadriceps femoris
   c. Hamstrings d. Peroneal muscles

Ans. is 'b' Quadriceps femoris

3. **A 82-year-old female with necrotic head of femur and bilateral osteoarthritis. What is the next step of management:**
   a. Uncemented total hip replacement
   b. Cemented total hip replacement
   c. Hemi-arthroplasty
   d. Observation

Ans. is 'b' Cemented total hip replacement

4. **Which is the most common joint involved in thalassemia?** *(Recent Pattern Question 2017)*
   a. Hip b. Knee
   c. Shoulder d. Ankle

Ans. is 'b' Knee

5. **Which of the following condition present as arthritis with conjunctivitis?** *(Recent Pattern Question 2017)*
   a. Reiter's syndrome
   b. Kaplan syndrome
   c. Pneumoconiosis
   d. Aspergillosis

Ans. is 'a' Reiter's syndrome

6. **Joint *not* involved in rheumatoid arthritis:**
   a. DIP b. PIP
   c. MC d. Wrist

Ans. is 'a' DIP

7. Which of the following is seen in Boutonniere's deformity:

a. Extension of PIP and DIP
b. Flexion of PIP and DIP
c. Flexion contracture of PIP and extension of DIP
d. Flexion of DIP and extension of PIP

Ans. is 'c' Flexion contracture of PIP and extension of DIP

8. All are seen in rheumatoid arthritis EXCEPT:

a. Boutonniere's deformity
b. Heberden nodes
c. Involvement of PIP
d. Swan neck deformity

Ans. is 'b' Heberden nodes

9. A 35-year-old female presented with MCP and PIP pain. Diagnosis:

a. Rheumatoid arthritis
b. Rheumatic fever
c. Gouty arthritis
d. Psoriatic arthritis

Ans. is 'a' Rheumatoid arthritis

10. Diagnosis of the picture given:

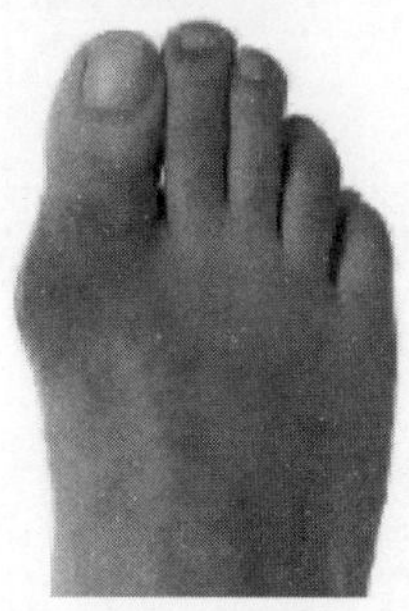

a. Osteoarthritis
b. Gouty arthritis
c. Rheumatoid arthritis
d. Pseudogout

Ans. is 'b' Gouty arthritis

11. Drug of choice for acute gouty arthritis:

a. Indomethacin
b. Allopurinol
c. Colchicine
d. Aspirin

Ans. is 'a' Indomethacin

12. Clutton's joint is seen in:

a. Early congenital syphilis
b. Late congenital syphilis
c. Tertiary syphilis
d. All of the above

Ans. is 'b' Late congenital syphilis

13. The following X-ray is diagnostic of which of the following condition:

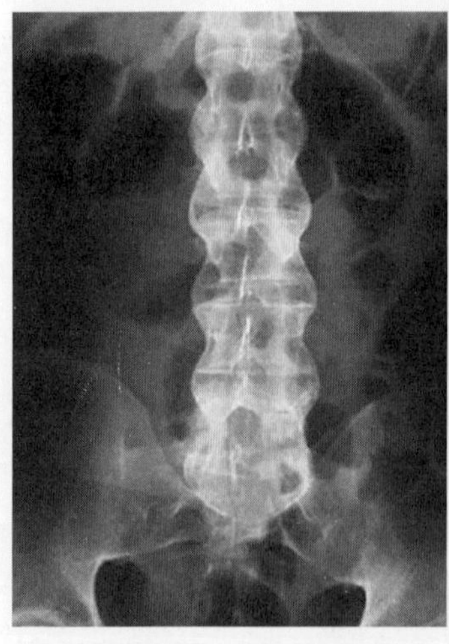
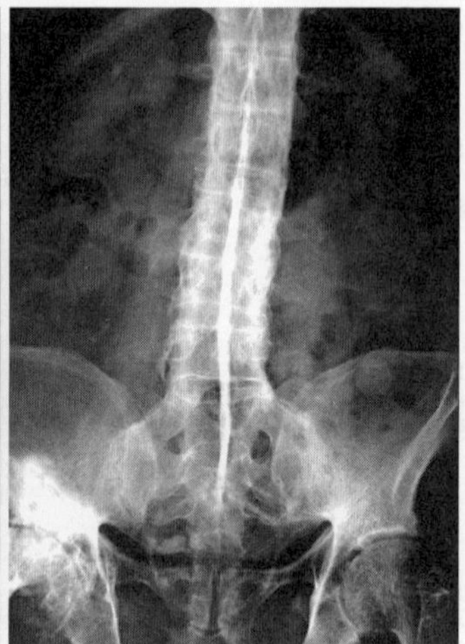

a. Rheumatoid arthritis
b. Ankylosing spondylitis
c. Hyperparathyroidism
d. Pagets disease

Ans. is 'b' Ankylosing spondylitis

14. Most common part of spine affected by rheumatoid arthritis is?

a. Lumbar spine
b. Thoracic spine
c. Cervical spine
d. Sacrum

Ans. is 'c' Cervical spine

15. Bone cement setting time is?

a. 30 seconds
b. 1-2 min
c. 8-10 min
d. >30 min

Ans. is 'c' 8-10 min

16. A 65-year-old male has been diagnosed osteoarthritis, feature or deformity seen is:

a. Swan neck deformity
b. Boutonniere deformity
c. Heberden's nodes
d. Opera glass deformity

Ans. is 'c' Heberden's nodes

17. Most common deformity seen in osteoarthritis is:

a. Genu valgum
b. Genu varum
c. Genu recurvatum
d. Triple knee deformity

Ans. is 'b' Genu varum

18. Joint spared in osteoarthritis:

a. DIP
b. PIP
c. Knee
d. Ankle

Ans. is 'd' Ankle

19. Most common joint involved in OA:

a. Knee
b. Elbow
c. Shoulder
d. Hip

Ans. is 'a' Knee

20. Main extensor of knee:

a. Gastrocnemius
b. Quadriceps femoris
c. Hamstrings
d. Peroneal muscles

Ans. is 'b' Quadriceps femoris

21. Which of the following seen in Boutonniere deformity:

a. Extension of PIP and DIP
b. Flexion of PIP and DIP
c. Flexion contracture of PIP and extension of DIP
d. Flexion of DIP and extension of PIP

Ans. is 'c' Flexion contracture of PIP and extension of DIP

22. Joint NOT involved in Rheumatoid Arthritis:

a. DIP　　b. PIP

c. MCP　　d. Wrist

Ans. is 'a' DIP

23. All are seen in Rheumatoid arthritis EXCEPT:

a. Boutonniere deformity　　b. Heberdens nodules

c. Involvement of PIP　　d. Swan neck deformity

Ans. is 'b' Heberdens nodules

24. Clutton's joint is seen in:

a. Early congenital syphilis

b. Late congenital syphilis

c. Tertiary syphilis

d. All of the above

Ans. is 'b' Late congenital syphilis

25. Case of a 60 years old man with severe knee pain limiting his daily activities. He has osteoarthritis on knee X-rays, his treatment is:

a. Cast application

b. Pain killers and physiotherapy

c. Brace

d. Total Knee Replacement

Ans. is 'd' Total Knee Replacement

26. All of the following are true regarding ankylosing spondylitis except:

a. Involvement of sacroiliac joint

b. Most of people are HLAB27 positive

c. 50% of patients may have urinary infection

d. Bamboo spine may be a radiological feature

Ans. is 'c' 50% of patients may have urinary infection

27. HLA B27 is commonly associated with which of the following:

a. Rheumatic fever　　b. Rheumatoid arthritis

c. Osteoarthritis　　d. Ankylosing spondylitis

Ans. is 'd' Ankylosing spondylitis

28. Iliac crest involvement is common in which condition:

a. Ankylosing spondylitis
b. Rheumatoid arthritis
c. Reiter's syndrome
d. Osteoarthritis

Ans. is 'a' Ankylosing spondylitis

29. All of the following are true regarding ankylosing spondylitis except: *(March 2010)*

a. Involvement of sacroiliac joint
b. Most of people are HLAB27 positive
c. 50% of patients may have urinary infection
d. Bamboo spine may be a radiological feature

Ans. is 'c' 50% of patients may have urinary infection

30. HLA B27 is commonly associated with which of the following: *(March 2010)*

a. Rheumatic fever
b. Rheumatoid arthritis
c. Osteoarthritis
d. Ankylosing spondylitis

Ans. is 'd' Ankylosing spondylitis

31. Most common joint involved in osteoarthritis in India: *(March 2009 (OA))*

a. Shoulder
b. Hip
c. Knee
d. Ankle

Ans. is 'c' Knee

32. Part of knee most commonly involved in osteoarthritis: *(March 2009 (OA))*

a. Medial compartment
b. Lateral compartment
c. Medial and lateral compartment
d. Patellofemoral compartment

Ans. is 'a' Medial compartment

33. Felty's syndrome is associated with which & of the following: *(September 2009 (RA))*

a. Osteoarthritis
b. Rheumatoid arthritis
c. Ankylosing spondylitis
d. Psoriatic arthritis

Ans. is 'b' Rheumatoid arthritis

34. Metacarpophalangeal joints are most commonly affected in: *(March 2005)*

a. Osteoarthritis
b. Psoriatic arthritis
c. Rheumatoid arthritis
d. Rheumatic fever

Ans. is 'c' Rheumatoid arthritis

35. Swan neck deformity is seen in: *(March 2013 (a, c, e))*

a. Ankylosing spondylitis
b. Rheumatoid arthritis
c. Osteoarthritis
d. Reiter's syndrome

Ans. is 'b' Rheumatoid arthritis

36. Joint LEAST involved in primary osteoarthritis: *(March 2013 (b, h))*

a. Hip
b. Trapeziometacarpal
c. Knee
d. Coracoclavicular

Ans. is 'd' Coracoclavicular

37. Crystals deposited in Pseudogout: *(March 2013 (d))*

a. Sodium biurate
b. Calcium oxalate
c. Calcium pyrophosphate
d. Amyloid

Ans. is 'c' Calcium pyrophosphate

38. Atlantoaxial subluxation is the most commonly seen manifestation of:

a. Rheumatoid arthritis
b. Septic arthritis
c. Ankylosing spondylitis
d. Spondylosis

Ans. is 'a' Rheumatoid arthritis

39. Most common Charcot's joint involved in diabetes mellitus are those of:

a. Knee
b. Foot
c. Ankle
d. Shoulder

Ans. is 'b' Foot

40. The classical deformity of rheumatoid hand is:

a. Trigger finger
b. Mallet finger
c. Swan-neck finger
d. None of the above

Ans. is 'c' Swan-neck finger

41. Earliest joint to be affected in ankylosing spondylitis is:

a. Hip joint
b. Shoulder joint
c. Sacroiliac joint
d. Elbow joint

Ans. is 'c' Sacroiliac joint

42. Heberden's nodes are the:

a. Subcutaneous nodules seen in RA
b. Swollen DIP classically in OA
c. Inflamed first MTP in gout
d. Osteophytes seem at the zygapophyseal joint in the spine

Ans. is 'b' Swollen DIP classically in OA

43. Example of syndesmosis joint is:

a. Tibiotalar joint
b. Tibiofibular joint
c. Elbow joint
d. Carpometacarpal joint

Ans. is 'b' Tibiofibular joint

44. Which is not included in diagnostic criteria's for rheumatoid arthritis:

a. Symmetric swelling
b. Morning stiffness
c. Positive Rheumatoid factor
d. Swelling of any 2 joints of the bodies

Ans. is 'd' Swelling of any 2 joints of the bodies

45. Heberden's nodes are the:

a. Subcutaneous nodules seen in RA
b. Swollen DIP classically in OA
c. Inflamed first MTP in gout
d. Osteophytes seem at the zygapophyseal joint in the spine

Ans. is 'b' Swollen DIP classically in OA

46. Iliac crest involvement is common in which condition: *(March 2007)*

a. Ankylosing spondylitis
b. Rheumatoid arthritis
c. Reiter's syndrome
d. Osteoarthritis

Ans. is 'a' Ankylosing spondylitis

47. In a patient with gouty arthritis, strongly birefringent needle-shaped crystals with negative elongation in syonvial fuid aspiration are composed of: *(September 2007)*

a. Monosodium urate
b. Calcium pyrophosphate
c. Homogentisic acid
d. Sodium pyrophosphate

Ans. is 'a' Monosodium urate

48. Urate crystals are deposited in small joints of the hands & feets in: *(September 2003)*

a. Gout
b. Still's disease
c. Retropharyngeal abscess
d. Ankylosing spondylitis

Ans. is 'a' Gout

49. Charcots/neuropathic joints are most commonly seen in:

a. DM
b. Syringomyelia
c. Leprosy
d. Rheumatoid arthritis

Ans. is 'a' DM

50. On X-ray, joint swelling & intra-articular 'calcification' appearance is seen in: *(September 2004)*

a. Osteopetrosis
b. Paget's disease
c. Rheumatoid arthritis
d. Charcot's joint

Ans. is 'd' Charcot's joint

51. Charcoat's joint includes all of the following EXCEPT: *(September 2012)*

a. Neurosyphilis
b. Leprosy
c. Diabetes
d. Arthrogryposis multiplex congenita

Ans. is 'd' Arthrogryposis multiplex congenita

52. The most common site of primary osteoarthrosis is: *(TAMILNADU 97)*

a. Hip joint
b. Knee joint
c. Ankle joint
d. Shoulder joint

Ans. is 'b' Knee joint

53. Bouchard's nodes are seen in: *(DPG Mar 09)*

a. Proximal IP joints
b. Distal IP joints
c. Sternoclavicular joints
d. Knee joint

Ans. is 'a' Proximal IP joints

54. Deformity most commonly seen in primary osteoarthritis of knee joint: *(NEET/DNB Pattern)*

a. Genu valgum
b. Genu recurvatum
c. Genu varus
d. Procurvatum

Ans. is 'c' Genu varus

55. Severe disability in primary osteoarthritis of hip is best managed by: *(PGI 95)*

a. Arthrodesis

b. Arthroplasty

c. McMurray's osteotomy

d. Intra-articular hydrocortisone and physiotherapy

Ans. is 'b' Arthroplasty

56. 40 years patient having arthritis of PIP and DIP along with carpometacarpal joint of thumb and sparing of wrist and metacarpophalangeal joint, most likely diagnosis is: *(AI 01, 00, AIIMS June 99. Dec 95)*

a. Rheumatoid arthritis

b. Osteoarthritis

c. Psoriatic arthritis

d. Pseudogout

Ans. is 'b' Osteoarthritis

57. Which joint is spared in Rheumatoid arthritis: *(NEET/DNB Pattern)*

a. MP joints of hand

b. DIP joints of finger

c. PIP joints of finger

d. Atlantoaxial joint

Ans. is 'b' DIP joints of finger

58. Swan-neck deformity is: *(AIIMS 2K, PGI 92)*

a. Flexion of Metacarpophalangeal joint and extension at interphalangeal joint

b. Extension at Proximal interphalangeal joint and flexion at Distal interphalangeal joint

c. Flexion at proximal interphalangeal joint and extension at distal interphalangeal joint

d. Extension at Metacarpophalangeal joint and flexion at interphalangeal joint

Ans. is 'b' Extension at Proximal interphalangeal joint and flexion at Distal interphalangeal joint

59. Butonniere deformity occur due to: *(PGI Dec 08)*

a. Flexion of Proximal interphalangeal joint
b. Flexion at Distal interphalangeal joint
c. Extension at Distal interphalangeal joint
d. Extension at Metacarpophalangeal joint
e. Flexion at Metacarpophalangeal joint

Ans. is 'a' Flexion of Proximal interphalangeal joint

60. Joint not involved in Rheumatoid arthritis according to 1987 modified ARA criteria? *(AIIMS Dec 08)*

a. Knee b. Ankle
c. Tarsometatarsal d. Metatarsophalangeal

Ans. is 'c' Tarsometatarsal

61. What is pathognomic feature of rheumatoid arthritis? *(AIIMS May 05)*

a. Rheumatoid factor
b. Rheumatoid nodule
c. Morning stiffness
d. Ulnar drift of fingers

Ans. is 'b' Rheumatoid nodule

62. In rheumatoid arthritis, pathology starts in the: *(AI 95)*

a. Articular cartilage b. Capsule
c. Synovium d. Muscles

Ans. is 'c' Synovium

63. Earliest radiological change in RA: *(NEET/DNB Pattern)*

a. Decreased joint space
b. Articular erosion
c. Periarticular osteopenia
d. Subchondral cyst

Ans. is 'c' Periarticular osteopenia

64. Ankylosing spondylitis is associated with: *(AI 99)*

a. HLA-B27 b. HLA-B-8
c. HLA-DW4/DR4 d. HLA-DR3

Ans. is 'a' HLA-B27

65. In ankylosing spondylitis, radiological change are first seen in: *(DPG 10)*

a. Sacroiliac joints
b. Intervertebral ligament
c. Vertebral bodies
d. Intervertebral discs

Ans. is 'a' Sacroiliac joints

66. Bamboo spine with sacroiliitis: *(NEET/DNB Pattern)*

a. Ankylosing spondylitis
b. RA
c. OA
d. Psoriatic arthritis

Ans. is 'a' Ankylosing spondylitis

67. Terminal interphalangeal joints of hands are commonly involved in: *(AI 93)*

a. Psoriatic arthropathy
b. Rheumatoid arthritis
c. Still diseases
d. Ankylosing spondylitis

Ans. is 'a' Psoriatic arthropathy

68. MC joint involved in Gout: *(AIIMS May 95)*

a. Knee
b. Hip
c. MP joint of the big toe
d. MP joint of thumb

Ans. is 'c' MP joint of the big toe

69. Specific test for gout is: *(AI 98, AIIMS Sept 96)*

a. Raised serum uric acid level
b. Raised uric acid in synovial fluid of joint
c. Raised urea level
d. Raised urease enzyme level

Ans. is 'b' Raised uric acid in synovial fluid of joint

70. Drug used in acute gout: *(NEET/DNB Pattern)*

a. Allopurinol
b. Probenecid
c. Colchicine
d. Sulfinpyrazone

Ans. is 'c' Colchicine

71. A lady presents with right knee swelling. Aspiration was done in which CPPD crystals were obtained. Next best investigation is: *(AIIMS May 10)*

a. ANA
b. RF
c. CPK
d. TSH

Ans. is 'd' TSH

72. Most common charcot's joints involved in diabetes mellitus are those of: *(AI 97)*

a. Shoulder
b. Ankle
c. Knee
d. Foot

Ans. is 'd' Foot

73. Joints of hand are not affected in: *(NEET/DNB Pattern)*

a. AS
b. RA
c. OA
d. Psoriatic arthritis

Ans. is 'a' AS

Chapter 16

Metabolic Disorders of Bone

There are four types of metabolic bone diseases.

a. ***Osteopenic diseases:*** These diseases are characterized by a generalized decrease in bone mass (i.e., loss of bone matrix), though whatever bone is there, is normally mineralized (e.g., osteoporosis).
b. ***Osteosclerotic diseases:*** There are diseases characterized by an increase in bone mass (e.g., fluorosis).
c. ***Osteomalacic diseases:*** These are diseases characterized by an increase in the ratio of the organic fraction to the mineralized fraction i.e., the available organic matter is undemineralized.
d. ***Mixed diseases:*** These are diseases that are a combination of osteopenia and osteomalacia (e.g., hyperparathyroidism).

Note:

- ***Rickets:*** Lack of adequate mineralization of growing bones.
- ***Osteomalacia:*** Lack of adequate mineralization of trabecular bone.
- ***Osteoporosis:*** Proportionate loss of bone volume and mineral.
- ***Scurvy:*** Defect in osteoid formation.

RICKETS AND OSTEOMALACIA

Increase in Osteoid Maturation Time

Osteoid matrix is secreted at normal rate but the mineralization is decreased (i.e., decrease in mineral apposition rate). This leads to increased osteoid maturation time. (Maturation of osteoid means mineralization of osteoid). Osteoid is increased in thickness, volume and total surface area. Bone tissue throughout skeleton is incompletely calcified and therefore softened. Rickets refers to condition where it occurs before closure of growth plates so that abnormalities of skeletal growth are superimposed.

Pathology

Hence osteoid is laid down irregularly with widened osteoid seams and osteoid islets may even persist down into the diaphysis. The new trabeculae are thin and weak (as bundle of collagen fibers instead of running parallel to haversian canal, coarse perpendicularly) and with joint loading the juxtaepiphyseal metaphysis becomes broad and cup shaped'.

A - **A**bdomen protuberant
B - **B**owing of bones (on weight bearing)
C - **C**ostochondral Junction prominent - (Rosary), **C**raniotabes (open fontanelles)
D - **D**iaphragm pull - Harrisons groove (Lateral indentation of chest due to pull of diaphragm on ribs)/**D**ouble Malleolus
E - **E**namel defect of teeth and delayed dentition
F - **F**orward sternum - Pigeon chest (Pectus carinatum)
G - **G**rowth plate - widening
H - **H**ypocalcemia causing **h**yper PTH
I - **I**rritability
J - **J**oint deformities - Genu Valgum/Genu Varum
K - **K**yphosis
L - **L**ooser's Zones
M - **M**ilestone delayed. Muscle Weakness
R - **R**ickets

Causes of Rickets

1. Vitamin D disorders
   - Nutritional
   - Secondary, malabsorption, decrease in liver (25) hydroxylase activity, CRF
   - VDDR Type I
     Deficiency of 1alpha hydroxylase
   - VDDR Type II
     End organ resistance to 1.25 (OH)2 Vitamin D3 (high prevalence of alopecia, ectodermal defects.)

2. Calcium deficiency
3. Phosphorus deficiency
4. Renal losses
   a. Fanconi syndrome
   b. Distal RTA
   c. X-linked dominant (commonest), autosomal dominant and Autosomal recessive are 3 varieties of hypophosphatemic Rickets - increase incidence of skeletal deformities, no hypocalcemia.
5. Tumor associated with rickets.
   - Soft tissues – Hemangiopericytoma
   - Bone Tumors – Non-ossifying fibroma, giant cell tumors, osteoblastoma, fibrous dysplasia, and neurofibromatosis.

	Calcium	Phosphate	ALP	PTH
Osteoporosis	Normal	Normal	Normal	Normal
Rickets/ osteomalacia	N or low	Low	High	High
Primary hyper-parathyroidism	High	Low	High	High
Paget's disease	Normal	Normal	High	Normal

"Hypophosphatemic rickets has normal PTH"

S. alkaline Phosphatase is an Index of Osteoblastic Activity

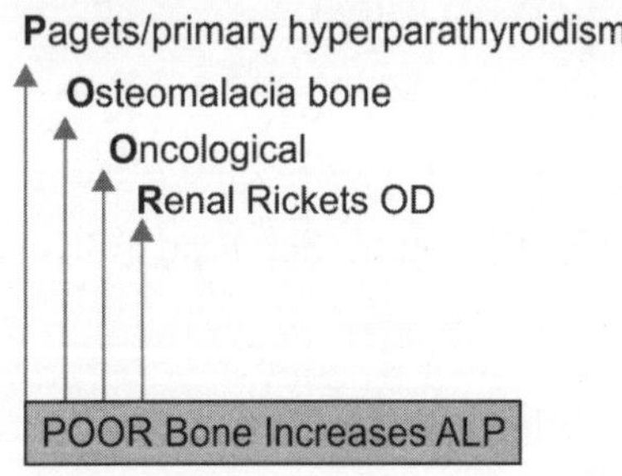

Normal-Osteoporosis, Multiple myeloma or Hypoparathyroidism (n or decrease).

RADIOGRAPHIC FINDINGS

- The characteristic feature of rickets are thickening and widening of growth plate (physis). Indistinct and hazy metaphysis that is abnormally wide (splaying) with cupping or flaring. (Brush like appearance).

  Bowing of diaphysis, with thinning of cortices.

  Looser's zone in 20%.
- Persistent hypocalcemia may cause secondary hyperparathyroidism.

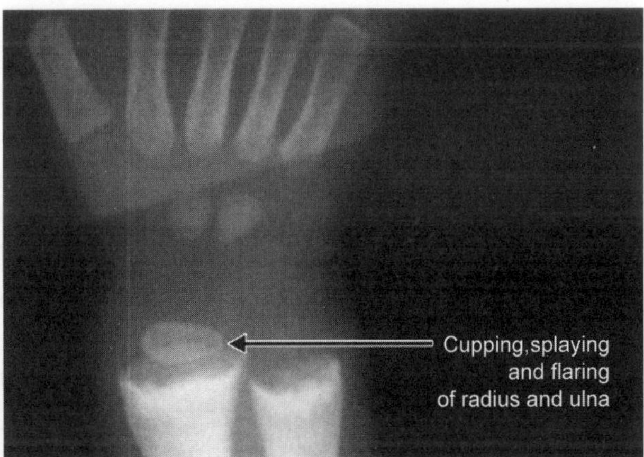

Fig. 16.1: Rickets

Therapy

1. Nutritional Rickets
   - 2 strategies for administration of vitamin D. Stoss therapy, 300,000–600,000 I.U. of vitamin D are administered orally or intramuscularly as 2–4 doses over 1 day. The alternative is daily high dose vitamin D, 2000 – 5000 I.U./day over 4–6 week followed by 400 I.U. Vitamin D/ Day and supplements of calcium for 2–4 months.

     Osteomalacia: Adult onset bone softening and muscle weakness. Low back and thigh pain, proximal muscle weakness. Triradiate pelvis, protrusio acetabular (acetabulum protrudes into pelvis due to bone softening when bilateral called as Otto Pelvis), Pseudofracture. There is waddling gait due to muscular weakness.

SCURVY

Scurvy: Deficiency of vitamin C, causing defect in osteoid formation.

Pathology

- Vitamin C is necessary for hydroxylation of lysine and proline to hydroxylysine and hydroxyproline, two aminoacids crucial for proper cross linking of triple helix of collagen. So deficiency causes failure of collagen synthesis or primitive collagen formation, throughout the body, including in blood vessels, predisposing to hemorrhage.
- In bones zone of proliferation is affected primarily.
- Hemorrhage, is capillary in origin and occurs from gums, alimentary tract, subcutaneous tissue, and bone especially at the most actively growing metaphysis and beneath periosteum.
- Haemorrhage and fractures are common, but attempts of repair are disordered. The provisional zone of calcification is weak leading to epiphyseal separations.
- Dysfunctional osteoblast (flat resembling fibroblast) causes failure of osteoid formation resulting in generalized osteoporosis.
- Chondroblast and mineralization is unaffected leading to persistence of calcified cartilage approaching metaphysis seen radiologically as opaque white line at junction of physis and metaphysis (Frankel's line).
- Osteoclasts are normal, thin and fragile trabeculae and cortices of bone are seen.
- Dentin formation in teeth is abnormal due to defective collagen.

Clinical Features

- It develops after 6 - 12 months of dietary deprivation thus not seen in neonates.
- Earliest features are restlessness, fretfulness, irritability, loss of appetite and failure to thrive.
- Gums may be spongy and bleeding.
- Subperiosteal haemorrhage is a distinct sign occuring most commonly in distal femur and tibia and proximal humerus, causing excruciating tenderness pain near the large joints. The child lies still to minimize pain or minimally move the affected limb (Pseudoparalysis) - **(Frogs Like Posture is attained by child)**

- Haemorrhage in soft tissue, joint, kidney, gut and petechiae may be seen.
- Anemia and impaired wound healing is seen.
- Beading of ribs at costochondral junction (Scorbutic Rosary).
- Systemic reaction (fever) is absent initially.

Note: In **R**ickets - Rosary is **R**ound and non-tender, and in **S**curvy it is **S**harp and tender.

Radiological Features

- Osteopenia (ground glass appearance) (1st sign) with thinning of cortex (Pencil thin cortex).
- Metaphysis may be deformed or fractured.
- Frankel's line (zone of provisional calcification increases in width and opacity) due to failure of resorption of calcified cartilage and stands Out compared to the severely osteopenic metaphysis.
- Scurvy line or scorbutic zone (Trummerfeld zone) is radiolucent transverse band adjacent to the dense provisional zone.
- Margins of the epiphysis appears relatively sclerotic, termed ringing of epiphyses or wimberger's sign (Ring sign) - Important.
- Lateral metaphyseal spur (Pelkan spur) at ends of metaphysis is produced by outward projection of zone of provisional calcification and periosteal reaction.
- Corner or angle sign is peripheral metaphyseal cleft.
- Subperiosteal haemorrhage.

Treatment: Vitamin C.

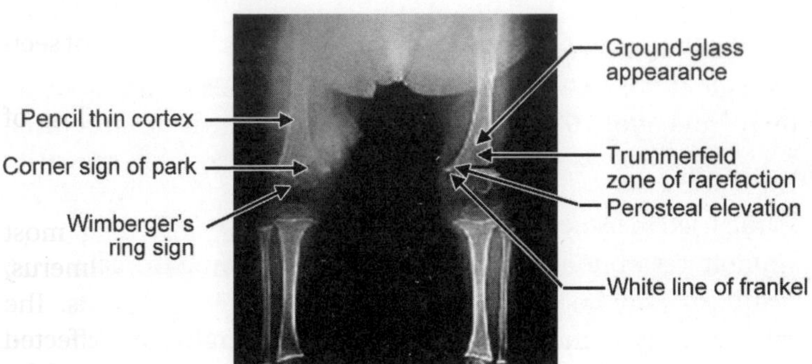

Fig. 16.2: Scurvy

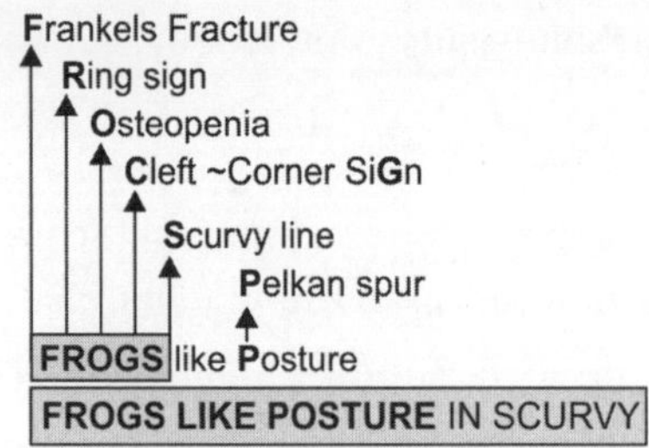

OSTEOPOROSIS

Osteoporosis is reduction in bone mass (density), i.e. there is quantitative decrease of units of bone formation but each unit has qualitatively normal configuration. So osteoporosis characteristically has normal calcium normal phosphate and normal alkaline phosphatase level.

Bone mineral density is measured by DEXA (Dual Emission X-ray Absorptiometry) Scan and it is matched to Dexa scan of **30** year old individual and **T** score is calculated.

WHO Classification.

- **T score 0 to -1 is normal**
- **T score -1 to -2.5 is osteopenia**
- **T score less than -2.5 is osteoporosis**
- **Osteoporosis with a fracture is severe osteoporosis**

The fractures that are most common (in decreasing order) are vertebral fracture, hip (neck femur) and lower end radius.

Most of the vertebral fractures are asymptomatic and are identified incidentally during radiograph for other purpose. Few of these present as backache of varying degree.

Upto age of 70, Colles' fracture is m.c. fracture in osteoporotic patient; and after 70 years age vertebral fracture is mc. fracture.

Treatment

1. Drug used in osteoporosis
   Inhibit resorption: Bisphosphonates, **Denosumab**, calcitonin, estrogen, SERMS, gallium nitrate.
2. Stimulate formation: **Teriparatide (PTH analogue)**, calcium, calcitriol, **fluorides**.
3. Both actions: Strontium Ranelate.

PAGET'S DISEASE/OSTEITIS DEFORMANS

It is characterized by excessive disorganized bone turnover that encompasses excessive osteoclastic activity initially followed by disorganized excessive new bone formation. It is the osteoclast that appears larger and irregular whereas osteoblast is relatively normal.

- The new bone formed is abnormal, very vascular and larger (deforms and fractures) than pre-existing bone which leads to cortical widening and contributes to the deformity.

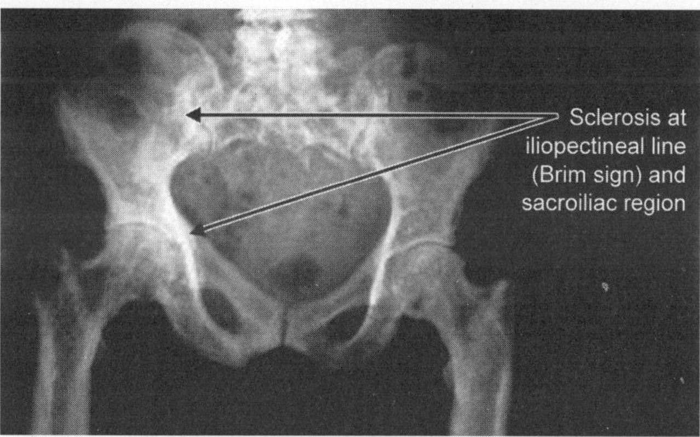

Fig. 16.3: X-ray pelvis: Paget's disease

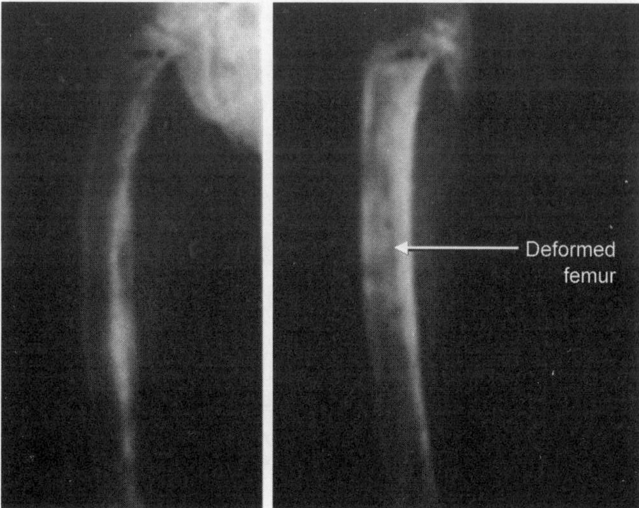

Fig. 16.4: X-ray femur: Pagets' disease

- The diagnostic histological feature of paget's disease is irregular areas of lamellar bone fitting together like a jigsaw with randomly distributed cement lines.
- It either occurs in one bone (monostotic Paget's disease) or multiple bones (polyostotic Paget's disease).

Etiology

- Genetic infection by paramyxovirus (measles and respiratory syncytial virus) has been linked.
- *Pathophysiology:* Increased bone resorption accompanied by accelerated bone formation is characteristic feature.
- Initial osteolytic phase involves prominent bone resorption and marked hypervascularization (Radiologically seen as advancing lytic wedge or **blade** of **grass lesion**) 2nd phase of active bone formation and resorption replaces normal lamellar bone with structurally weak woven bone that bend, bow and fracture easily.
- In 3rd sclerotic (burnt out) phase, bone resorption declines progressively and leads to hard, dense, less vascular pagetic or **mosaic bone.**

Clinical Features

- Most people are asymptomatic.
- The sites most commonly involved are - **pelvis**, tibia, followed by skull, spine, clavicle and femur.
- **Affects men more commonly.**
- **Pain is most common presenting symptom.**
- Limb look bent and feels thick, and skin is unduly warm due to high vascularity hence the name osteitis deformans. Skull show frontal bossing and platybasia.

Complications

1. Pagetoid bone lacks the strength of normal bone. As a result it deforms and fractures more easily.
2. Cranial nerve ~ 2nd, 5th, 7th, 8th palsy is seen.
3. Nerve compression and spinal stenosis is seen.
4. ***Deafness due to nerve compression > otosclerosis***
5. High output cardiac failure, Hypercalcemia (if immobilized).
6. Osteosarcoma (<1%) cases (poorest prognosis).

7. Steal syndrome i.e. blood is diverted from internal organs to skeleton system, may lead to cerebral ischemia and spinal claudication.
8. Osteoarthritis of hip and Knee is common.

Diagnosis

A. Serum calcium and phosphate levels are usually normal.
B. Increased marker of bone formation (e.g. S. alkaline phosphatase and S. Osteocalcin) **(ALP levels are used for monitoring pagets)**
C. Increased markers of bone resorption
   Serum and urinary deoxypyridinoline, N-telopeptide and C-telopeptide
   Urinary hydroxyproline
   - Urinary deoxypyridinoline (24 hours assessment) is most valuable.

Radiological Features

- Long bone X-ray shows deformity, enlargement or expansion of bone with cortical thickening coarsening of trabecular markings and lytic and sclerotic changes.
- Skull X-ray reveal "cotton wool" or osteoporosis circumscripta, thickening of diploic area. **Increasing Hat Size!**
- Vertebral cortical thickening at superior and inferior end plates creates a picture frame vertebrae and diffuse sclerosis causing ivory vertebrae
- Pelvic radiograph show sclerotic iliopectineal line (Brim sign), fusion or disruption of sacroiliac joints, etc.

Treatment

Indications are

A. To control symptoms of active disease as bone pain, fracture, neurological complications or pain from radiculopathy or arthropathy.
B. To decrease local blood flow and minimize operative blood loss in patients undergoing surgery.
C. To decrease hypercalciuria
D. To decrease complications -When site of involvement involves weight bearing bones, skull, vertebral bodies and major joints.

E. Bisphosphonates are drug of choice and calcitonin is used to relieve pain.
F. Surgery is done for pathological fracture, osteoarthritis, nerve entrapment and spine decompression.

OSTEOPETROSIS

Marble Bone Disease or Albers Schonberg Disease

Etiopathology

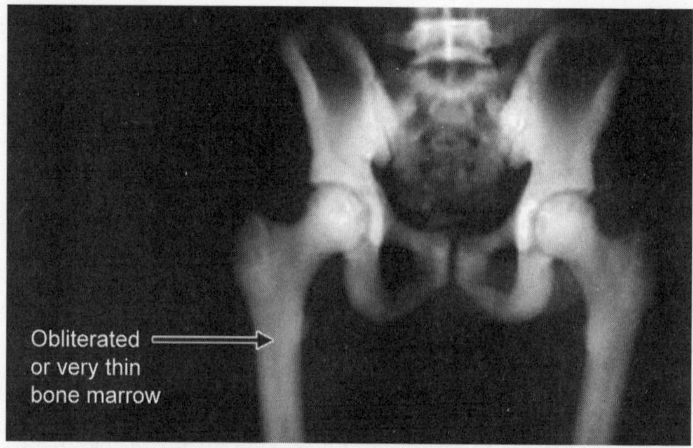

Fig. 16.5: Osteopetrosis

- It is a diaphyseal dysplasia characterized by failure of bone resorption due to functional deficiency of osteoclast. The bone contains increased number of osteoclasts but these don't resorb bone as evidenced by absence of ruffled borders and clear zones and are unable to respond to PTH. Due to functional deficiency of osteoclasts, calcified chondroid (cartilage) and primitive woven bone persists down into metaphysis and diaphysis leading to osteosclerosis and increased brittleness of bones (marble bone disease)
- Inheritance depends on form of disease: Malignant osteopetrosis (congenital form) is autosomal recessive (AR, 11q 13) and late onset Osteopetrosis tarda (adolescence /adult form) is AD (1P 21).
- Intermediate form is AR.

Clinical Presentation

- Autosomal dominant, benign or tarda osteopetrosis is often diagnosed in adult asymptomatic patients. It may present with mild anemia, pathological fractures premature osteoarthritis, and rarely osteomyelitis of mandible.
- Autosomal recessive malignant (congenital) osteopetrosis clinically presents at birth or in early infancy because of Obliteration of marrow cavity by bony overgrowth resulting in inability of bone marrow to participate in hematopoiesis. Pancytopenia develops resulting in abnormal bleeding, easy bruising, progressive anemia, and failure to thrive.
- Severe infections esp. Mandible.
- Extramedullary hematopoiesis causing hepatosplenomegaly.
- Cranial nerve palsies (Bony Overgrowth of Cranial Foramen) 2nd, 7th and 8th - blindness and deafness.
- Fragile brittle bones.
- Pathological fractures.
- Radiological hallmark is increased radiopacity of bones. There is no distinction between cortical and cancellous bone, because intramedullary canal is filled with bone.
- Endobones (os-in-os or bone with in bone appearance) and rugger jersey spine.
- Treatment is bone marrow transplant.

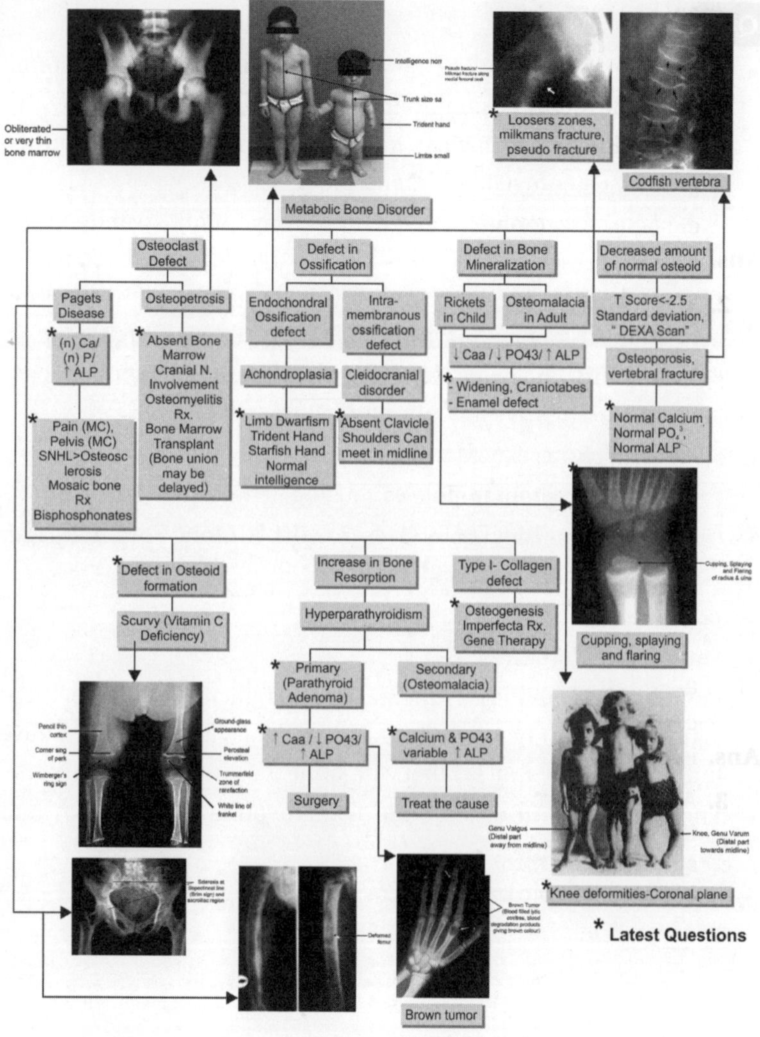

Obliterated or very thin bone marrow
Intelligence nor
Trunk size sa
Trident hand
Limbs small
Loosers zones, milkmans fracture, pseudo fracture
Codfish vertebra
Metabolic Bone Disorder
Osteoclast Defect
Defect in Ossification
Defect in Bone Mineralization
Decreased amount of normal osteoid
Pagets Disease
Osteopetrosis
Endochondral Ossification defect
Intra-membranous ossification defect
Rickets in Child
Osteomalacia in Adult
T Score<-2.5 Standard deviation, " DEXA Scan"
(n) Ca/ (n) P/ ↑ ALP
Absent Bone Marrow Cranial N. Involvement Osteomyelitis Rx. Bone Marrow Transplant (Bone union may be delayed)
Achondroplasia
Cleidocranial disorder
↓ Caa / ↓ PO43/ ↑ ALP
Osteoporosis, vertebral fracture
- Widening, Craniotabes - Enamel defect
Pain (MC), Pelvis (MC) SNHL>Osteosclerosis Mosaic bone Rx Bisphosphonates
Limb Dwarfism Trident Hand Starfish Hand Normal intelligence
Absent Clavicle Shoulders Can meet in midline
Normal Calcium Normal PO4, Normal ALP
Cupping, Splaying and Flaring of radius & ulna
Defect in Osteoid formation
Increase in Bone Resorption
Type I- Collagen defect
Scurvy (Vitamin C Deficiency)
Hyperparathyroidism
Osteogenesis Imperfecta Rx. Gene Therapy
Cupping, splaying and flaring
Primary (Parathyroid Adenoma)
Secondary (Osteomalacia)
Pencil thin cortex
Corner sing of park
Wimberger's ring sign
Ground-glass appearance
Periosteal elevation
Trummerfeld zone of rarefaction
White line of frankel
↑ Caa / ↓ PO43/ ↑ ALP
Calcium & PO43 variable ↑ ALP
Surgery
Treat the cause
Genu Valgus (Distal part away from midline)
Knee, Genu Varum (Distal part towards midline)
Knee deformities-Coronal plane
Sclerosis at iliopectineal line (Brim sign) and sacroiliac region
Deformed femur
Brown Tumor (Blood filled lytic cavities, blood degradation products giving brown colour)
Brown tumor
* Latest Questions

QUESTIONS

1. **Which of the following is the management of postmenopausal women with osteoporosis:**

   (Recent Pattern Question 2018)

   a. Raloxifene
   b. Tamoxifen
   c. Bisphosphonates
   d. Calcitonin

Ans. is 'c' Bisphosphonates

2. **X-ray wrist and hand of a child is given below. There is prominent cupping and widening of growth plage. What is the diagnosis:** *(Recent Pattern Question 2017)*

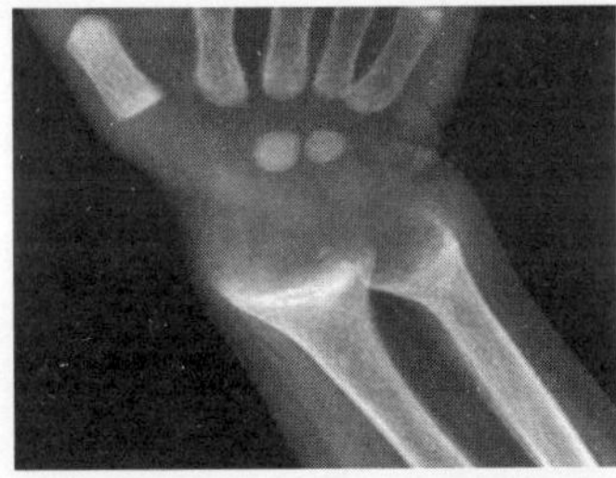

   a. Fluorosis
   b. Plumbism
   c. Vitamin C deficiency
   d. Vitamin D deficiency

Ans. is 'd' Vitamin D deficiency

3. **A case of young patient is presented to you with knee pain, irritability and gum bleeding. Upon X-ray of leg, cortex is significantly thin with a white line at the metaphysis. What could be possible cause?**

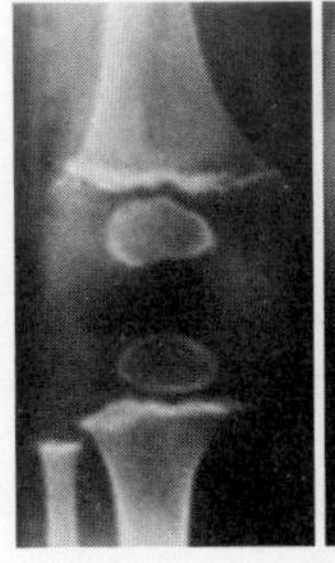
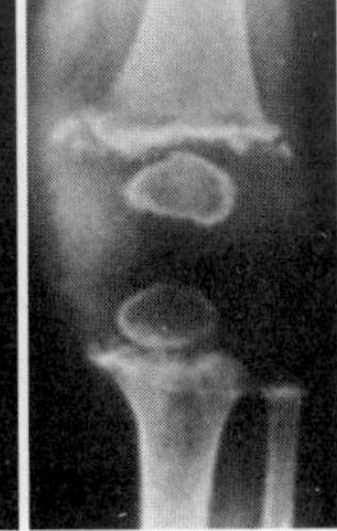

   a. Fluorosis
   b. Rickets
   c. Scurvy
   d. Caffey's disease

Ans. is 'c' Scurvy

4. A 7-year-old boy presented double medial malleolus. X-ray was performed. What is the treatment?

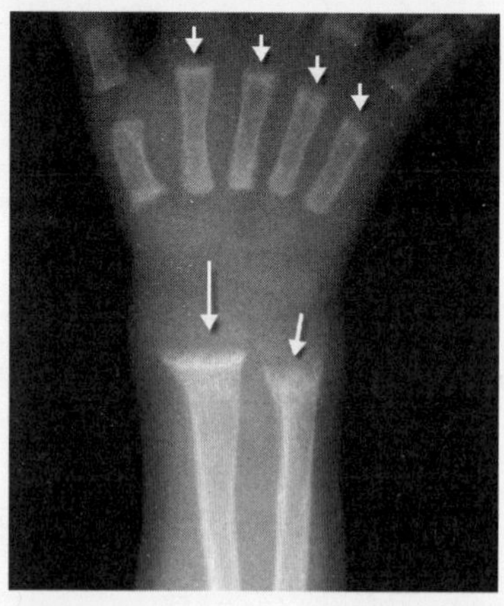

a. Vitamin B
b. Vitamin C
c. Vitamin D
d. Vitamin E

Ans. is 'c' Vitamin D

5. A child from a small village of Bihar has long bone pain, is weak and lethargic and on examination he has bow legs. The X-ray reports shows increase in bone density, osteophytes and dysmorphic joint space. Possible diagnosis is:

a. Fluorosis
b. Rickets
c. Scurvy
d. Caffey's disease

Ans. is 'a' Fluorosis

6. Stoss therapy is used for:

a. Scurvy
b. Vitamin D deficiency rickets
c. Vitamin D Resistant rickets
d. Paget's disease

Ans. is 'b' Vitamin D deficiency rickets

7. All of the following are true about osteomalacia *except*:

a. Vitamin D deficiency
b. Proximal myopathy
c. Raised serum calcium
d. Bone biopsy shows increased demineralized bone matrix

Ans. is 'c' Raised serum calcium

8. Most common cause of bone disease especially in women in India:

a. Steroid-induced osteoporosis
b. Nutritional deficiency
c. Paget's disease
d. Sarcoidosis

Ans. is 'b' Nutritional deficiency

9. Loosers zones are seen in:

a. Osteoporosis
b. Osteomalacia
c. Osteosarcoma
d. TB Spine

Ans. is 'b' Osteomalacia

10. Short 4th and 5th metacarpal is seen in:

a. Pseudohypoparathyroidism
b. Hyperparathyroidism
c. Hyperthyroidism
d. Hypothyroidism

Ans. is 'a' Pseudohypoparathyroidism

11. Stoss therapy is used for?

a. Scurvy
b. Rickets
c. Vitamin D resistant rickets
d. Hyperparathyroidism

Ans. is 'b' Rickets

12. Which of the following is not true about Scurvy:

a. Vitamin C is deficient
b. Wimberger ring sign is seen
c. Defect in hydroxylation of collagen is seen
d. Cupping of bony ends is seen

Ans. is 'd' Cupping of bony ends is seen

13. A patient with Genu varum with beading of costochondral junction with widening of bony ends in most likely to be:

a. Rickets
b. Scurvy
c. Fluorosis
d. Hyperparathyrodism

Ans. is 'a' Rickets

14. All are diagnostic features of osteomalacia *except*:

a. Increased serum calcium *(March 2011)*

b. Increased alkaline phosphatase

c. Proximal myopathy

d. Looser's zone

Ans. is 'a' Increased serum calcium

15. Serum alkaline phosphate is normal in: *(September 2009)*

a. Osteosarcoma b. Osteomalacia

c. Multiple myeloma d. Malnutrition

Ans. is 'c' Multiple myeloma

16. "Marble Bone" appearance is seen in: *(March 2009)*

a. Osteomalacia b. Osteopetrosis

c. Rickets d. Osteoporosis

Ans. is 'b' Osteopetrosis

17. Wimberger 'Ring sign' is seen in: *(September 2003) (scurvy)*

a. Scurvy b. Congenital syphilis

c. Gaucher's disease d. All of the above

Ans. is 'a' Scurvy

18. Arachnodactyly/spider fingers is seen in: *(March 2003)*

a. Down's syndrome b. Turner's syndrome

c. Marfan's syndrome d. All of the above

Ans. is 'c' Marfan's syndrome

19. All statements are true for osteomalacia *except*:

a. Looser's zone on X-ray *(March 2012)*

b. Commoner in females

c. Raised serum calcium

d. Muscular weakness

Ans. is 'c' Raised serum calcium

20. Codfish vertebrae are seen in: *(March 2004)*

a. Osteopetrosis b. Osteoporosis

c. Morquio syndrome d. All of the above

Ans. is 'b' Osteoporosis

21. Regarding osteoporosis, all of the following statements are true *except*: *(March 2012)*

a. Raised alkaline phosphatase
b. DEXA scan is helpful
c. Reduced bony matrix
d. Codfish appearance on X-ray

Ans. is 'a' Raised alkaline phosphatase

22. Sub-periosteal bone absorption is best seen in:

a. Radius
b. Metacarpals
c. Phalanges
d. Ulna

Ans. is 'c' Phalanges

23. Osteopetrosis results due to defective:

a. Osteoblasts
b. Osteoclasts
c. Bone collagen
d. Phosphate deposition in trabecular bone

Ans. is 'b' Osteoclasts

24. "Bone within bone" appearance is classically seen in:

a. Osteomalacia
b. Osteopetrosis
c. Renal osteodystrophy
d. Vitamin C deficiency

Ans. is 'b' Osteopetrosis

25. In epiphyseal injuries, the line of epiphyseal separation is:

a. Zone of cartilage cell
b. Zone of provisional calcification
c. Zone of resting cartilage cell
d. Zone of proliferating cartilage cell

Ans. is 'd' Zone of proliferating cartilage cell

26. Relentless pain in a patient with Paget's disease indicates:

a. Malignant degeneration
b. Pathological fracture
c. Secondary osteoarthritis
d. All of the above

Ans. is 'd' All of the above

27. The disease that results in deficient hydroxylation of the pro-alpha chains of collagen is known as:

a. Scurvy

b. Rickets

c. Ehlers-Danlos syndrome

d. Marfan's syndrome

Ans. is 'a' Scurvy

28. Serum alkaline phosphate is normal in:

a. Osteosarcoma b. Osteomalacia

c. Multiple myeloma d. Malnutrition

Ans. is 'c' Multiple myeloma

29. Albers schonberg disease is: *(PGI June 2k 98)*

a. Osteopetrosis b. Osteoporosis

c. Osteochondritis d. Osteomalacia

Ans. is 'a' Osteopetrosis

30. Looser's zone is present in:

a. Multiple myeloma b. Osteomalacia

c. Pseudoparathyroidism d. Osteoporosis

Ans. is 'b' Osteomalacia

31. All of the following are seen in rickets *except*:

a. Frankels line

b. Widening of epiphysis-diaphysis distance

c. Cupping and splaying of metaphysis

d. Rarefaction

Ans. is 'a' Frankels line

32. All of the following are true about rickets *except*:

a. Craniotabes b. Rachitic rosary

c. Knock-knees d. Hypertonia

Ans. is 'd' Hypertonia

33. Rachitic rosary is a feature of: *(March 2013 (c))*

a. Rickets b. Scurvy

c. Osteomalacia d. Osteoporosis

Ans. is 'a' Rickets

34. Most common cause of genu valgum in children is:

a. Osteoarthritis
b. Rickets
c. Pager's disease
d. Rheumatoid arthritis

Ans. is 'b' Rickets

35. Osteomalacia is due to: *(NEET/DNB Pattern)*

a. Vitamin C deficiency
b. Vitamin D deficiency
c. Vitamin E deficiency
d. None

Ans. is 'b' Vitamin D deficiency

36. Decreased mineralization of Epiphyseal plate in a growing child is seen in: *(Al 2K)*

a. Rickets
b. Osteomalacia
c. Scurvy
d. Osteoporosis

Ans. is 'a' Rickets

37. Which of the following is a persistant biochemical marker of rickets? *(AI 98)*

a. S.Ca++
b. S. Alkaline phosphatase
c. S. Acid phosphate
d. S. phosphate

Ans. is 'b' S. Alkaline phosphatase

38. Radiological features of rickets include: *(PGI Dec 05)*

a. Narrowing of epiphysis
b. Cupping of metaphysis
c. Ricketic rosary
d. Pelkan's spur

Ans. is 'b' Cupping of metaphysis

39. A 67-year-old man on biochemical analysis found to have three fold rise of level of serum alkaline phosphatase that of upper limit of norm value during a routine checkup but serum calcium and phosphorous concentration and liver function test results and normal. He is asymptomatic. The probable cause is: *(AIIMS 99)*

a. Multiple myeloma
b. Paget's disease of bone
c. Primary hyperparathyroidism
d. Osteomalacia

Ans. is 'c' Primary hyperparathyroidism

40. A young patient presents with enlargement of costocondral junction and with the white line of Fraenkel at the metaphysis. The diagnosis is:

a. Scurvy b. Rickets
c. Hyperparathyroidism d. Osteomalacia

Ans. is 'a' Scurvy

41. Brown Tumor is seen in: *(AI 10, 06)*

a. Hypothyroidism
b. Hyperthyroidism
c. Hypoparathyroidism
d. Hyperparathyroidism

Ans. is 'd' Hyperparathyroidism

42. Absence of lamina dura in the alveolus occurs in: *(DPG Mar 09)*

a. Rickets
b. Osteomalacia
c. Deficiency of Vitamin C
d. Hyperparathyroidism

Ans. is 'd' Hyperparathyroidism

43. Paget's disease after 10 years develops: *(NEET/DNB Pattern)*

a. Osteosarcoma b. Fibrous cortical defect
c. Osteoid osteoma d. Ankylosing spondylitis

Ans. is 'a' Osteosarcoma

44. Most common site of osteoporosis: *(NEET/DNB Pattern)*

a. Humerus b. Vertebrae
c. Scapula d. Flat bones

Ans. is 'b' Vertebrae

45. "Trident hand seen in: *(AIIMS Dec 98)*

a. Achondroplasia
b. Mucopolysaccharidosis
c. Diaphyseal achiacia
d. Cleido-cranial dysostosis

Ans. is 'a' Achondroplasia

46. Mode of inheritance for achondroplasia is: *(PGI 96)*

a. Autosomal dominant

b. Autosomal recessive

c. X-linked dominant

d. X-linked recessive

Ans. is 'b' Autosomal dominant

47. Osteogenesis imperfecta is defect in: *(PGI 98)*

a. Bone

b. Calcification

c. Cartilage

d. Collagen

Ans. is 'd' Collagen

Chapter 17

Pediatric Orthopedics

LEGG-CALVE-PERTHES DISEASE/ OSTEOCHONDRITIS DEFORMANS JUVENILIS/COXA PLANA

It can be defined as osteonecrosis of the proximal femoral epiphysis in a growing child caused by poorly understood (non-genetic) factors.

Pathogenesis

Clinical Presentation

- 4 to 8 years of age
- Most frequent symptom is limp that is exacerbated by activity and alleviated with rest.
- 2nd most frequent complaint is pain.
- Later on most movements are full, but abduction (especially in flexion) is nearly always limited and usually internal rotation also. **When the hip is flexed it may go into obligatory external rotation (catterall's sign or axis deviation) and knee points towards axilla.** (Normally goes towards mid-clavicular region)

Head at Risk sign have been described for perthes

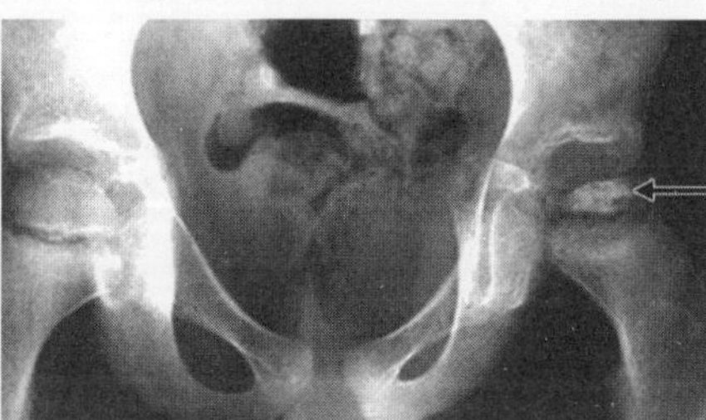

Fig. 17.1: Perthes disease

Investigation

MRI is the investigation of choice.

Management

The main aim of treatment is containment of femoral head in acetabulum. Non-surgical containment is achieved by orthotic braces All braces abduct the affected hip, most allow for hip flexion, and some control rotation of the limb. Broomstick or petrie cast issued.

Surgical containment is achieved through (1) Femoral varus derotation osteotomy, (2) Chiari osteotomy and cheilectomy (surgically removing protruding fragments of femoral head usually antero lateral).

Slipped Capital Femoral Epiphysis

During a period of rapid growth, **due** to weakening of upper femoral physis and shearing stress from excessive body weight, there is upward and anterior movement of femoral neck on the capital epiphysis. So **the epiphysis is located primarily posteriorly and medially relative to the femoral neck**.

Aetiology

- The cause is unknown in vast majority of patients.
- Many of the patients are either **fat and sexually immature** or excessively **thin and tall.**
- Endocrinopathies such as **Hypothyroidism** (most common)
- **Growth hormone** excess caused by growth hormone deficiency conditions treated by growth hormone administration.
- Chronic renal failure (Hyperparathyroidism)
- Primary **hyperparathyroidism**
- Pan hypopituitarism associated with intracranial tumors
- Craniopharyngioma
- MEN 2 B
- Turner's syndrome
- Klinefelters syndrome
- Rubinstein Taybi syndrome
- Prior pelvic irradiation
- Many a times it presents in **growth spurt**.

Pathogenesis and Pathology

Slip occurs through **hypertrophic zone of growth plate** classically in obese hypogonadal male (adiposogenital syndrome).

Clinical Picture

- An adolescent child (boys 13–15 and girls 11–13) typically overweight or very thin and tall presents with pain some times and Antalgic limp, with the affected side held in a position of increased external rotation, (turning out of leg). Restriction of internal rotation, abduction and flexion.
- **A classical sign is tendency of thigh to rotate in to progressively more external rotation, as the affected hip is flexed called as** Axis deviation. (Similar to Perthes).
- Chondrolysis **(Destruction of Cartilage) and** avascular necrosis **are possible complications.**

Investigation

A line drawn tangential to superior femoral neck **(klein's line)** on AP view will intersect a portion the lateral capital epiphysis normally. With typical posterior displacement of capital epiphysis this line will intersect a smaller portion of the epiphysis or not at all **trethowans sign.**

MRI is useful investigation for diagnosis.

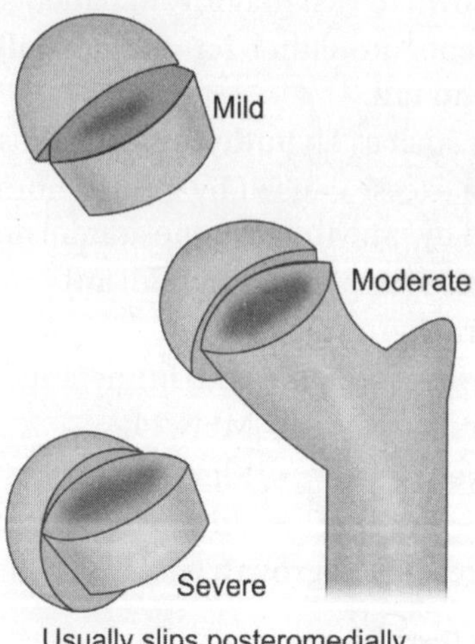

Fig. 17.2: Slipped capital femoral epiphysis

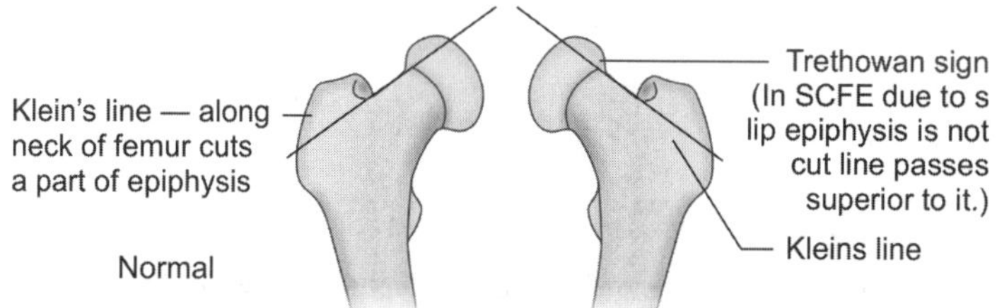

Fig. 17.3: Radiological diagnosis of slipped capital femoral epiphysis

Treatment

SCFE is usually a progressive disease that requires prompt surgical treatment. Acute slips, if unstable may be gently reduced before fixation but there are chances of AVN.

Developmental Dysplasia of Hip (DDH)—Shallow Acetabulum

DDH is failure of maintenance of femoral head due to malformations of acetabulum or femur. **Twin pregnancy does not increase the risk.**

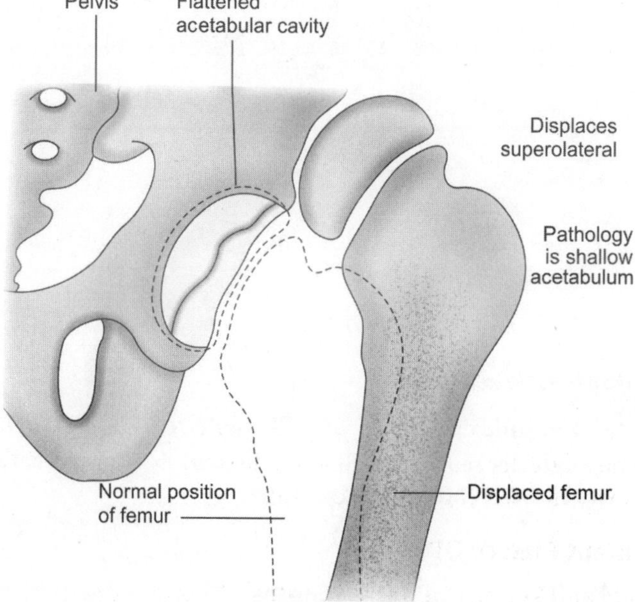

Fig. 17.4: DDH

Clinical Diagnosis

BAAHARLO! "DAD" i.e. Barlow's test - Dislocation By Adduction (DAd).

This in Barlows we dislocate hip joint.

IInd part – Now the hip is abducted and pulled. This will cause 'clunk' indicating reduction of hip.

Some consider only 1st part as Barlow's test

- Ortolani's Test – the first two alphabets **O** and **R** (Ortolani for Reduction) and for Reduction we do abduction of hip.
- It is similar to 2nd part of Barlow's test
- Short limb as shown by - Higher buttock folds, Galeazzi or Allis sign is lowering of knee on affected side in a lying child with hip and knees flexed.
- Trendelenburg's test, telescopy and vascular sign of Narath are positive.

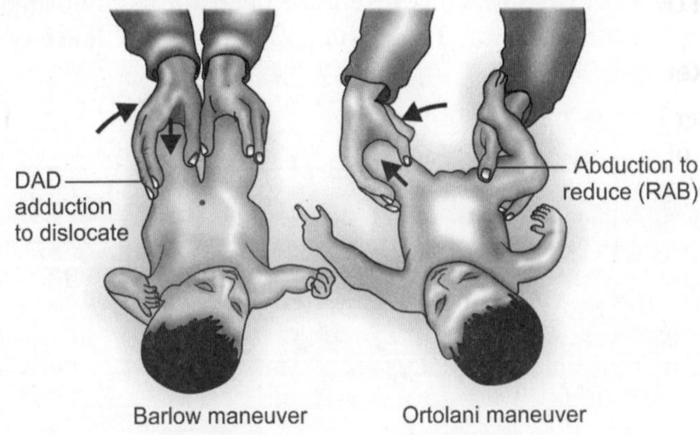

Fig. 17.5: Test for DDH

Radiological Features

- **Acetabular index increases and CE angle reduces in DDH.**
- **Alpha angle decreases and Beta angle increases with increasing severity in DDH (Measured on USG).**

Treatment Plan of DDH

Neonate and Young Child (1-6 months)-Closed reduction, Pavlik harness

6–18 months—open reduction is carried out

18–36 months

Open reduction + femoral rotation osteotomy ± pelvic osteotomy

Walking Child (3–6 years)

Open reduction (anterolateral approach) and femoral shortening with **Acetabular reconstruction procedure**: (Salter's, Chiari's pelvic displacement and Pemberton osteotomy).

6–10 years: treatment should be avoided (fear of AVN), in bilateral DDH, in unilateral same as above.

>11 years: in cases of painful hips due to Osteoarthritis, THR may be done (but should be delayed till skeletal maturity).

Congenital dislocation of knee-hyper extension (genu recurvatum) is the most common presentation Genu valgum - the commonest cause of genu valgum (knock knee) is idiopathic >rickets.

Note: Usually OA Causes Varum/RA Valgum.

Rocker Bottom Foot

Rocker bottom foot, is a foot with a convex plantar surface with an apex of convexity at the talar head is due to wrong correction of CTEV or congenital vertical talus.

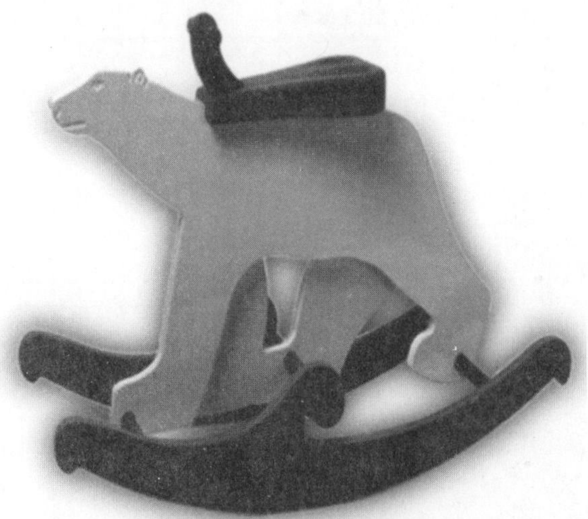

Fig. 17.6: Rocker bottom

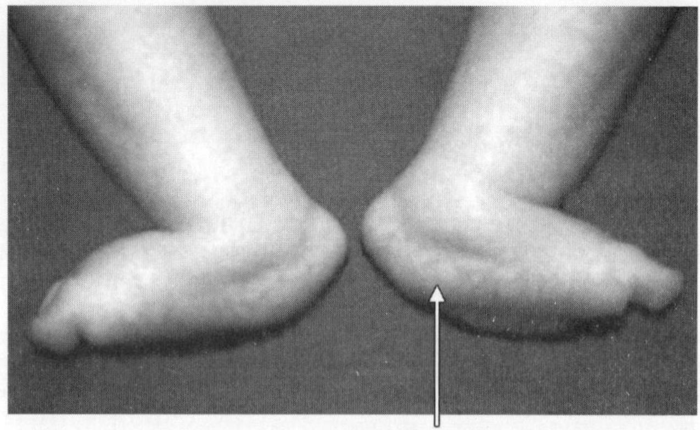

Fig. 17.7: Rocker bottom foot

Club Foot/Congenital Talipes Equinovarus (CTEV)

Pirani/Dimeglio scoring is for CTEV

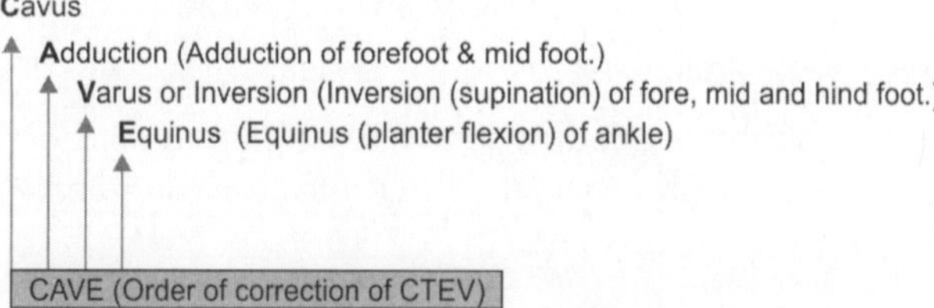

- Kites angle – AP view talocalcaneal angle.
- Normal value is 20 to 40 degrees (decreased in CTEV)

Club stick to play
golf CTEV foot
resembles it so
called as club foot.

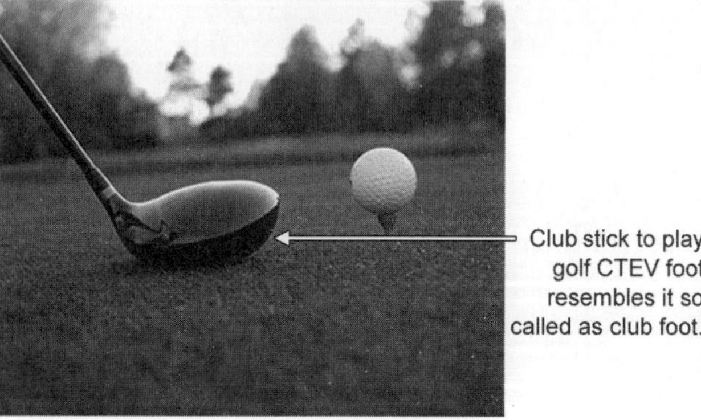

Fig. 17.8: Club

Most Common Relapse in CTEV— Adduction

Treatment is

<1 year cast (starting from birth)

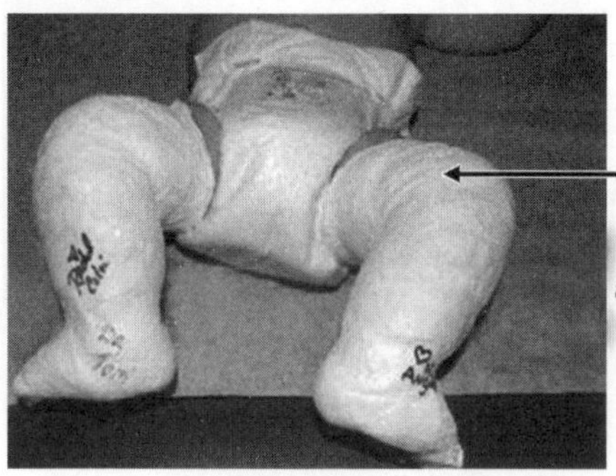

Fig. 17.9: Above knee CTEV cast

1 to 3 years Soft tissue release-Posteromedial soft tissue release (Turco)

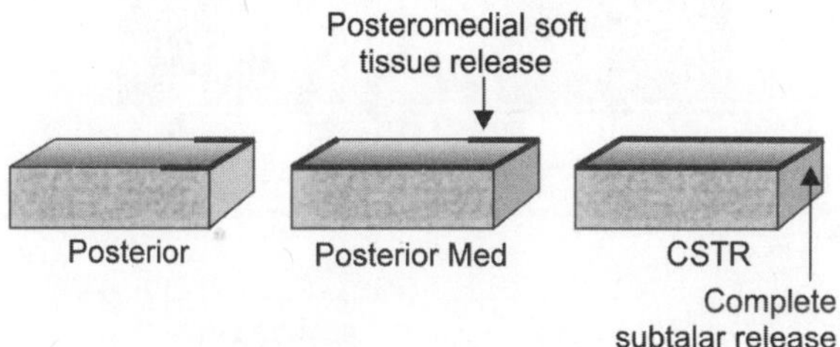

Fig. 17.10: Soft tissue releases

But in children older than 3 years of age lateral column shortening procedures are often performed in conjunction with posteromedial soft tissue release.

3–8 years

Soft tissue release together with shortening of lateral side of foot by.

Evan-Dillwyn Procedure (i.e., resection and fusion of calcaneo cuboid joint).

Dwyer's osteotomy of calcaneum is done to correct calcaneal varus in >5 years.

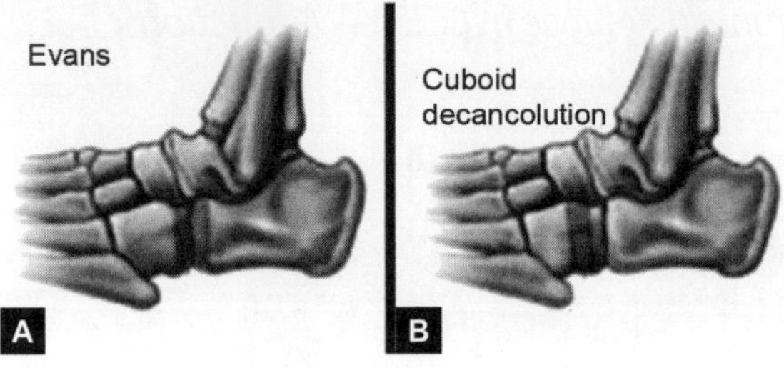

Figs. 17.11A and B: Lateral column shortening

8–10 years

Wedge Tarsectomy is done as deformity is more and requires multiple bones to be removed.

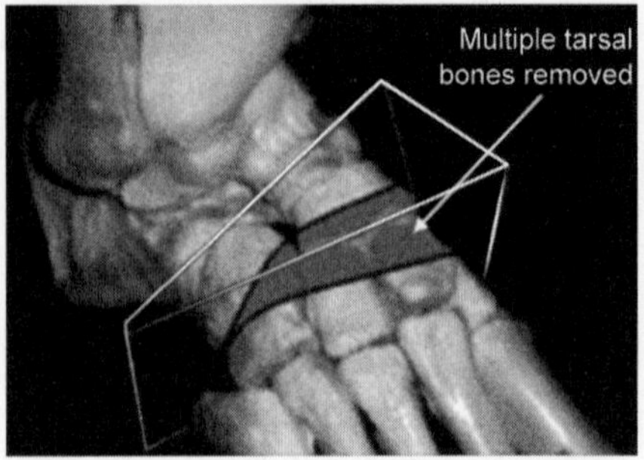

Fig. 17.12: Wedge tarsectomy (8–10 years)

>10 years

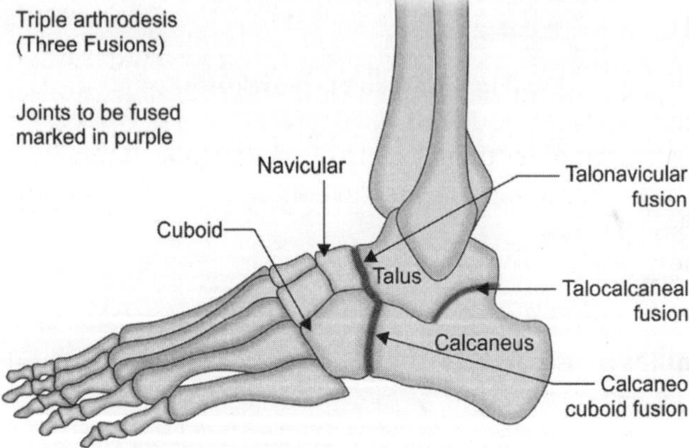

Fig. 17.13: Triple arthrodesis (>10 years)

Triple arthrodesis is necessary for recurrent **or** persistent clubfoot deformity in older children (chronic cases). It is best done at >10 years of age when foot growth is complete and the bones are ossified to achieve good fusion.

It involves fusion of three joints: **TN - Talo-Navicular; TC – Talo-Calcaneal; CC – Calcaneo-Cuboid.** *(AIPG 2008)*

Fractures in Children

The immature skeleton has several unique properties that affect the management of injuries in children.

These properties include thicker periosteum, soft bones, an increased resiliency to stress, an increased potential to remodel, shorter healing times, and the presence of a physis. This can lead to some characteristic fracture patterns in pediatric population.

Greenstick fracture – break in single cortex of the bone

Plastic deformation – bend of a bone without a break

- Distal radius and ulna is the most common site of fracture in children accounting for nearly a quarter of fracture.
- Forearm fractures in pediatric population are best treated by manipulation and cast
- 2nd in frequency is Hand injury
- 3rd in frequency are elbow injuries amongst them supracondylar fracture humerus are most common and
- 4th common is clavicle fracture
- Please remember that Clavicle is the most common fractured bone in adults and during birth.

*Dislocations and comminuted fractures are rare in children.

Remember most common joint to dislocate in adults is shoulder but in children is elbow.

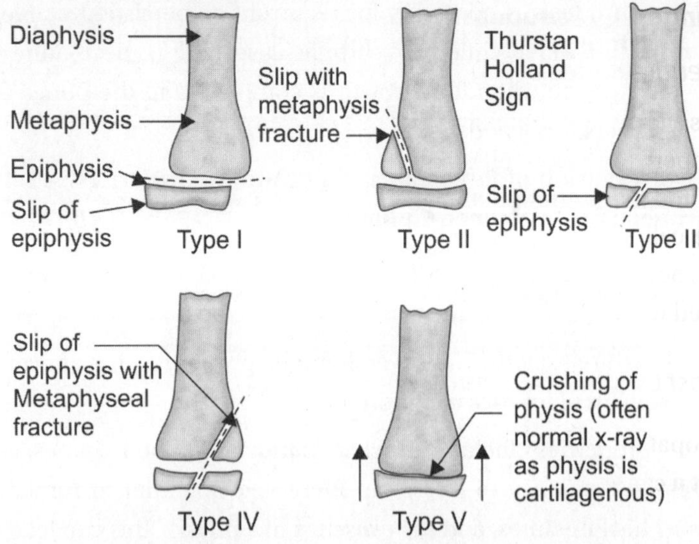

Fig. 17.14: Salter-Harris classification for epiphyseal injury

Remodeling Potential in Children

Remodeling of bone is best (maximum) for metaphyseal angulation deformity and least (worst) for diaphyseal rotation deformity.

Salter-Harris classification is used for epiphyseal injuries in children.

Thurstan holland sign is type 2 epiphyseal injury

Radial club hand –mannux valgus deformity

The radius is absent so is thumb causing lateral deviation of hand called as mannux valgus deformity.

Klippel-Feil Syndrome

Klippel-Feil Syndrome is congenital fusion of one or more cervical vertebrae presenting with classical triad of low hair line, short 'web' neck (prominence of trapezius muscle), and limited neck motion seen in 50% cases.

Note: Usually Skeletal disorders are Autosomal Dominant and Inborn errors of metabolism are Autosomal Recessive.

Congenital Pseudoarthrosis

Pseudoarthrosis

It is a false joint that may develop after a fracture that has not united properly due to inadequate immobilization. If a nonunion allows for too much motion along the fracture gap, the central portion of the callus undergoes cystic degeneration and the luminal surface can actually become lined by synovial like cells, creating a false joint filled with clear fluid- known as pseudoarthrosis.

Most Common Cause of Pseudoarthrosis

Idiopathic > Neurofibromatosis (NF- 1) – **(Actually an association, not a cause)**

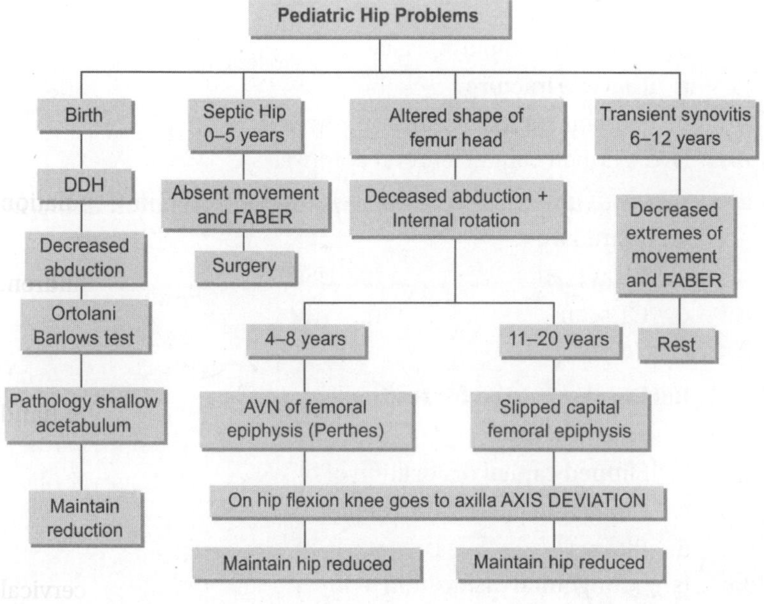

QUESTIONS

1. **The triad of triple arthrodesis includes all *except*:** *(Recent Pattern Question 2018)*
   a. Calcaneocuboid joint
   b. Talonavicular joint
   c. Tibiotalar joint
   d. Subtalar joint

Ans. is 'c' Tibiotalar joint

2. **Most common joint dislocation in pediatric population:** *(Recent Pattern Question 2017)*
   a. Wrist
   b. Sternoclavicular
   c. Elbow
   d. Hip

Ans. is 'c' Elbow

3. **Trethowan sign is used for diagnosis of:** *(Recent Pattern Question 2017)*
   a. Talar fracture
   b. Congenital hip dysplasia
   c. Clavicle fracture
   d. Slipped capital femoral epiphysis

Ans. is 'd' Slipped capital femoral epiphysis

4. **Investigation for screening congenital dislocation of hip in an infant is:**
   a. X-ray
   b. USG
   c. CT scan
   d. MRI

Ans. is 'b' USG

5. **Barlow test is used for testing:**
   a. Talar fracture
   b. Slipped capital dislocation of hip
   c. Congenital dislocation of hip
   d. Rickets

Ans. is 'c' Congenital dislocation of hip

6. **Which ligament is involved in Pes-planus?**
   a. Spring ligament
   b. Deep transverse ligament
   c. Long & short plantar ligament
   d. Deltoid ligament

Ans. is 'a' Spring ligament

7. Vertical talus is associated with:

a. Congenital flat foot
b. Ankle dislocation
c. Talus fracture
d. Pes cavus

Ans. is 'a' Congenital flat foot

8. Fairbank's triangle is seen in?

a. Tibia vara
b. Genu valgum
c. Hip fracture
d. Coxa vara

Ans. is 'd' Coxa vara

9. Charlie Chaplin gait is seen in?

a. Congenital coxa vara
b. Tibial torsion
c. Genu valgus
d. CDH

Ans. is 'b' Tibial torsion

10. Spot diagnosis for foot deformity?

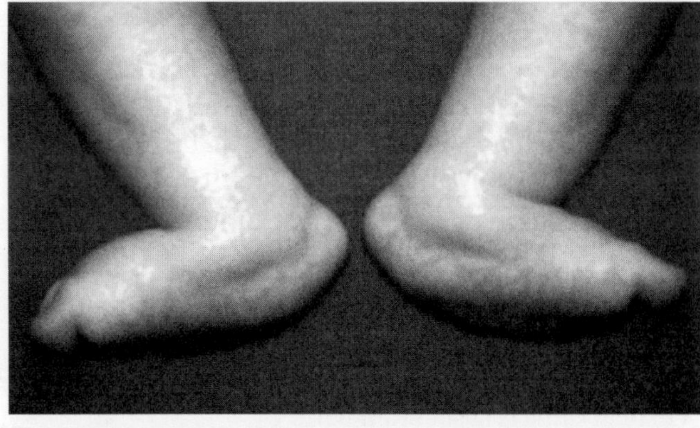

a. CTEV
b. Congenital vertical talus
c. Rocker bottom foot
d. Pes Cavus

Ans. is 'c' Rocker bottom foot

11. Multiple fractures in a child at birth are seen in which condition:

a. Battered baby syndrome
b. Hypoparathyroidism
c. Resistant rickets
d. Osteogenesis imperfecta

Ans. is 'd'Osteogenesis imperfecta

12. Gower's sing is seen in:

a. Guillain-Barre syndrome
b. Duchene muscular dystrophy
c. Congenital myopathy
d. All of the above

Ans. is 'b' Duchene muscular dystrophy

13. Radial club hand/Manus valgus is due to: *(March 2013 (f))*

a. Absence of ulna
b. Absence of radius
c. Carpal bones absent
d. Absence of humerus

Ans. is 'b' Absence of radius

14. Perthe's disease is osteochondritis of the epiphysis of the: *(March 2013 (g))*

a. Capitulum
b. Lunate
c. Femoral head
d. Calacaneal tuberosity

Ans. is 'c' Femoral head

15. Thurstan Holland sign/fragment is seen in: *(March 2004)*

a. Oblique fracture of lower 1/3rd humerus
b. Reverse oblique fracture of intertrochanteric femur
c. Salter-Harris type II fracture
d. Coronal fracture of femoral condyles

Ans. is 'c' Salter-Harris type II fracture

16. Vertical talus is associated with:

a. Congenital flat foot
b. Rocker bottom foot
c. Talus fracture
d. Pes cavus

Ans. is 'b' Rocker bottom foot

17. Barlow test & ortolani test is done for:

a. CTEV b. CDH
c. Both d. None

Ans. is 'b' CDH

18. Best method of treatment of fracture of both bones of the forearm in a 5 year old child is:

a. Open reduction and fixation with rush nails
b. External fixation
c. Manipulation and POP cast application
d. Massages

Ans. is 'c' Manipulation and POP cast application

19. Which of the following is the most convenient method for treatment of fracture shaft femur in children less than 2 years of age?

a. Open reduction and internal fixation
b. Reduction and A/K POP casing
c. Gallows traction
d. External fixation

Ans. is 'b' Reduction and A/K POP casing

20. All the following are useful in diagnosis of congenital dislocation of the hip *except*:

a. Ortolani's test
b. Barlow's test
c. Slocum test
d. Galeazzi or Ali's test

Ans. is 'c' Slocum test

21. Epiphyseal plate fractures are classified by:

a. Herring's classification
b. Salter-Harris classification
c. Garden's classification
d. Pauwel's classification

Ans. is 'b' Salter-Harris classification

22. Complication of humeral lateral epicondyle fracture is:

a. Non-union
b. Tardy ulnar nerve palsy
c. Cubitus valgus deformity
d. All of the above

Ans. is 'a' Non-union

23. Idiopathic scoliosis is an:

a. Laterals contracture of the spine
b. Rotation of the spine
c. Laterals curvature with rotation of spine
d. Flexion deformity of the spines

Ans. is 'c' Laterals curvature with rotation of spine

24. Triple arthrodesis is:

a. Arthrodesis of subtalar joint
b. Arthrodesis of talonavicular joint
c. Arthrodesis of calcaneocuboid joint
d. All of the above

Ans. is 'd' All of the above

25. Which joint is not fused in triple arthrodesis?

a. Tibiotalar
b. Talocalcaneal
c. Talonavicular
d. Calcaneonavicular

Ans. is 'a' Tibiotalar

26. Congenital talipes equinovarus deformity includes all of the following *except*: *(March 2010)*

a. Eversion
b. Forefoot adduction
c. Forefoot cavus
d. Equinus

Ans. is 'a' Eversion

27. In Triple Arthrodesis, which of the following joint is NOT fused?

a. Calcaneocuboid
b. Talonavicular
c. Tibiotalar
d. Subtalar

Ans. is 'c' Tibiotalar

28. Triple arthrodesis does not involve: *(September 2010)*

a. Calcaneocuboid Joint
b. Talanovicular Joint
c. Talocalcaneal Joint
d. Tibiotalar Joint

Ans. is 'd' Tibiotalar joint

29. Causes of Torticollis are all *except*:

a. Sternomastoid tumor
b. Neurogenic
c. Ocular causeSaint compensation
d. Frozen shoulder
e. Tonsilitis

Ans. is 'd' Frozen shoulder

30. Duchenne's muscular dystrophy affects which group of muscles commonly? *(September 2009)*

a. Calf muscles
b. Shoulder muscles
c. Forearm muscles
d. Respiratory muscles

Ans. is 'a' Calf muscles

31. In Duchennes muscular dystrophy, calf muscle is: *(September 2009)*

a. Hypertrophied
b. Atrophied
c. Pseudoatrophied
d. Pseudohypertrophied.

Ans. is 'd' Pseudohypertrophied

32. The ideal treatment of bilateral idiopathic clubfoot in a newborn is: *(AI 06)*

a. Manipulation by mother
b. Manipulation and Dennis Brown splint
c. Manipulation and casts
d. Surgical release

Ans. is 'c' Manipulation and casts

33. A newborn child presents with inverted foot and the dorsum of the foot cannot touch the anterior tibia. The most probable diagnosis is: *(AIIMS Nov 10)*

a. Congenital vertical talus
b. Arthrogryposis multiplex
c. CTEV
d. Flat foot

Ans. is 'c' CTEV

34. Green stick fracture is? *(NEET/DNB Pattern)*

a. Fracture in adults
b. Complete fracture
c. Incomplete fracture
d. Fracture spine

Ans. is 'c' Incomplete fracture

35. An 8-year-old boy with a history of fall from 10 feet height complains of pain in the right ankle. X-ray taken at that time are normal without any fracture line. But after 2 years he developed a calcaneovalgus deformity. The diagnosis is: *(AIIMS May 01)*

a. Undiagnosed malunited fracture
b. Avascular necrosis talus
c. Tibial epiphyseal injury
d. Ligamentous injury of ankle joint

Ans. is 'c' Tibial epiphyseal injury

36. Perthe's disease is: *(AIIMS May 94, NEET/DNB Pattern)*

a. Fracture of femoral shaft Pattern)
b. Osteochondritis of femoral epiphysis
c. Infarction of femoral head
d. Fracture dislocation of femoral neck

Ans. is 'b' Osteochondritis of femoral epiphysis

37. Slipped capital femoral epiphysis is seen most commonly in which age group? *(NEET/DNB Pattern)*

a. Infants
b. Adolescents
c. Old age
d. Childhood

Ans. is 'b' Adolescents

38. Commonest deformity in congenital dislocation of hip:
(PGI 97)

a. Small head of femur
b. Angle of torsion
c. Decreased neck shaft angle
d. Shallow acetabulum

Ans. is 'd' Shallow acetabulum

39. Provocative Test for detecting CDH?
(MH 10, NEET/DNB Pattern)

a. Peterson test
b. Barlow test
c. Perkin's test
d. Von Rosen tests

Ans. is 'b' Barlow test

Chapter 18

Osteochondritis Dissecans

- It is a poorly understood disorder, which leads to softening and separation of a portion of joint surface; resulting in development of small segment of necrotic bone in joint.
- Knee (lower- lateral part of medial femoral condyle) is the most commonly affected joint. Elbow (capitulum) is 2nd common.

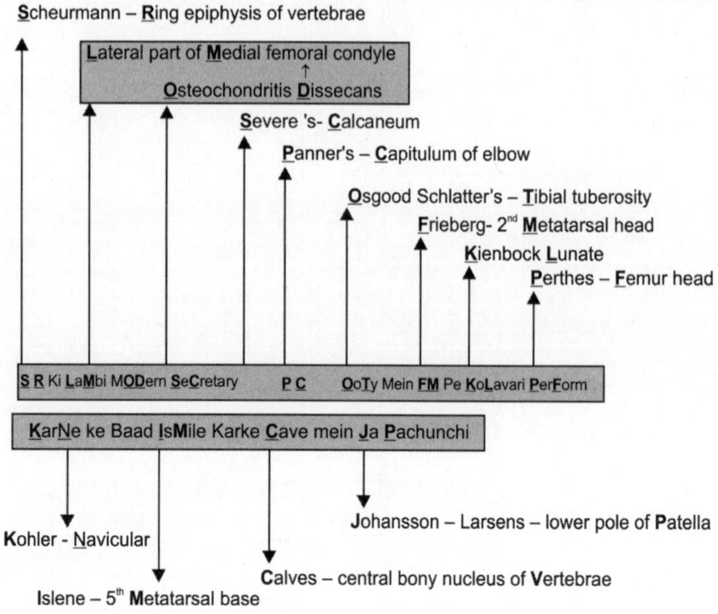

Scheurmann – Ring epiphysis of vertebrae

Lateral part of Medial femoral condyle
↑
Osteochondritis Dissecans

Severe 's- Calcaneum

Panner's – Capitulum of elbow

Osgood Schlatter's – Tibial tuberosity

Frieberg- 2nd Metatarsal head

Kienbock Lunate

Perthes – Femur head

S R Ki **L**a**M**bi M**OD**ern **S**e**C**retary **P C** **O**o**T**y Mein **FM** Pe **K**o**L**avari **P**er**F**orm

Kar**N**e ke Baad **I**s**M**ile Karke **C**ave mein **J**a **P**achunchi

Kohler - **N**avicular

Islene – 5th **M**etatarsal base

Calves – central bony nucleus of **V**ertebrae

Johansson – Larsens – lower pole of **P**atella

QUESTIONS

1. Osgood-Schlatter's disease involves?

a. Tibial tuberosity b. Femoral condyle
c. Lateral malleolus d. Medial malleolus

Ans. is 'a' Tibial tuberosity

2. Kienbock disease involves: *(2018)*

a. Capitate b. Lunate
c. Talus d. Trapezoid

Ans. is 'b' Lunate

3. Kienbock disease is avascular necrosis of:

a. Scaphoid b. Trapezoid
c. Trapezium d. Lunate

Ans. is 'd' Lunate

Chapter 19

Avascular Necrosis

Avascular necrosis: It is death of a bone due to poor blood supply.

Most common sites of avascular necrosis

Head of femur (most common)

Incidence of AVN in fracture neck Femur -Subcapital > transcervical > basicervical.

(Most important-supply of femoral head lateral epiphyseal branch of medial circumflex femoral artery supplies femoral head).

Scaphoid (proximal pole AVN)-because blood supply distal to proximal.

Talus (Body)

Lunate

Note: Think AVN as an answer if mentioned any disease for which steroids are given, e.g. Nephrotic syndrome or pemphigus vulgaris.

Investigation of choice: MRI

Treatment: 1. Core De-compression to decrease the pressure inside the bone

2. Re-vascularisation of the bone using muscle pedicle graft.

3. Joint replacement.

QUESTIONS

1. Kienbock disease is avascular necrosis of:

a. Scaphoid
b. Trapezoid
c. Trapezium
d. Lunate

Ans. is 'd' Lunate

2. **Aseptic necrosis is common in:** *(March 2007, September 2010)*

a. Scaphoid b. Calcaneum
c. Cuboid d. Trapezium

Ans. is 'a' Scaphoid

3. **Best diagnostic modality to diagnose avascular necrosis is:**

a. MRI scan b. CT scan *(March 2007)*
c. X-ray d. USC

Ans. is 'a' MRI Scan

4. **AVN is seen in:** *(March 2013 (a))*

a. Navicular fracture b. Talus fracture
c. Calcaneal fracture d. Cuboid fracture

Ans. is 'b' Talus fracture

5. **Aseptic necrosis is commoner in fractures of:** *(September 2011)*

a. Calcaneum b. Scaphoid
c. Cuboid d. Trapezium

Ans. is 'b' Scaphoid

6. **Avascular necrosis is commoner in:** *(March 2012)*

a. Cuboid b. Calcaneum
c. Navicular d. Talus

Ans. is 'd' Talus

7. **Avascular necrosis can be a possible sequelae of fracture of all of the following bones, *except*:**

a. Femur neck b. Scaphoid
c. Talus d. Calcaneum

Ans. is 'd' Calcaneum

8. **All the following are causes of avascular necrosis of the femoral head *except*:**

a. Alcoholism
b. Steroid therapy
c. Patient on renal dialysis
d. Unmatched blood transfusion

Ans. is 'd' Unmatched blood transfusion

9. A 45-year-old was given steroids after renal transplant. After 2 years he had difficulty in walking and pain in both hips. Which one of the following is most likely cause: *(AI 05)*

a. Primary osteoarthritis

b. Avascular necrosis

c. Tuberculosis

d. Aluminum toxicity

Ans. is 'b' Avascular necrosis

10. After chronic use of steroids severe pain in right hip with immobility is due to: *(NEET/DNB Pattern)*

a. Avascular necrosis
b. Perthes disease
c. Hip dislocation
d. Osteoarthritis

Ans. is 'a' Avascular necrosis

Chapter 20 Complete Revision of Orthopedics for MCI (FMGE)

Orthopaedics means straight child and the term was coined by Nicolas Andry.

Periosteal reaction in acute osteomyelitis can be seen at day 7 to day 10.

Avascular necrosis appears as cold areas on bone scan

Developmental dysplasia of hip or Congenital dislocation of hip – MRI>USG is investigation of choice.

Paronychia is most common infection of hand it is infection of nail bed of fingers and is caused by *Staphylococcus aureus.*

Felon or whitlow is infection of pulp space of finger, organism causing it is *Staphylococcus aureus.*

Most common organism causing hematogenous osteomyelitis is *Staphylococcus aureus.*

Most common route of spread of osteomyelitis is blood and most common location is metaphysis.

Tom smith arthritis is septic arthritis of hip in infancy

Broadies abscess is subacute osteomyelitis

Commonest location of Tuberculosis in musculoskeletal system is Spine (Pott's spine) and involvement is paradiscal

Commonest route of spread of tuberculosis to spine is hematogenous.

Commonest symptom of Pott's spine is pain and tuberculosis can have night cries.

Earliest sign in X-ray in T.B spine is straightening of spinal curves.

Monoarticular involvement is seen in tubercular arthritis

Tuberculosis Hip stage of synovitis there is flexion Abduction and external rotation at hip (FABER)

Triple deformity (Posterior subluxation, flexion and external rotation) of knee is a complication of tuberculosis of knee.

Caries sicca is a characteristic feature of Tuberculosis of shoulder

Spina ventosa is tubercular dactylitis

Most common cause of bony ankylosis is pyogenic arthritis

Tuberculosis of spine causes bony ankylosis

Fibrous ankylosis is seen in tubercular arthritis

ORTHOPAEDICS ONCOLOGY

- Chondroblastoma is epiphyseal tumor
- Osteosarcoma is metaphyseal tumor
- Most common sarcoma of bone in children is Ewing's sarcoma
- Shepherd crook deformity is seen in Fibrous dysplasia
- Soap bubble appearance is seen in GCT>Adamantinoma
- Mottled calcification is seen in Chondrosarcoma
- Sunray/Sun burst appearance is seen in osteosarcoma usually
- Onion peel appearance is seen in Ewing's sarcoma
- Solitary bone cyst is seen in Upper end of humerus and it is the most common cause of pathological fracture in child
- Aneurysmal bone cyst is seen in lower limbs (Tibia)
- Osteoid osteoma there is night pain relieved on taking salicylates (aspirin)
- Fibrous dysplasia is premalignant
- Upper end fibula GCT is treated by excision
- Adamantinoma is a common tumor of tibia
- Lower metaphysis of tibia intramedullary tumor in 15 year child is most likely osteosarcoma.
- Radiation induced sarcoma is osteosarcoma
- Ewings sarcoma is diaphyseal and most common age group is 2nd decade
- Ewing's is highly radiosensitive bone tumor but its treatment of choice is surgical excision and chemotherapy.
- Chondrosarcoma is common in flat bones and upper end of femur
- Physalipharous cells are seen in Chordoma
- Punched out lytic lesions are seen in multiple myeloma

- Multiple myeloma has high serum calcium, high ESR and normal alkaline phosphatase.
- Most common bone tumors and tumor of spine is secondaries (metastasis)
- Osteoblastic secondaries are seen in prostate
- Meningioma does not cause spinal cord compression

TRAUMATOLOGY

- Order of resuscitation is Airway, Breathing and Circulation
- Most common bone to fracture on face is nasal bone
- Most common site of fracture of mandible is neck of condyle
- Fracture and dislocation of lateral clavicle is treated surgically.
- Commonest type of shoulder dislocation is anterior
- Duga's test and Hamilton ruler test is for anterior dislocation
- Bankart's lesion is anterior tear of glenoid labrum seen in recurrent anterior dislocation.
- Hill-Sachs lesion is seen in recurrent anterior dislocation
- Anterior constraints prevent posterior shoulder dislocation
- Posterior dislocation is more common in convulsions and electric shock
- Electric bulb sign is seen in shoulder dislocation
- Luxatio erecta is inferior dislocation of shoulder
- Nerve commonly injured in shoulder dislocation is axillary nerve
- Axillary nerve supplies over regimental badge area
- Static Stabilizer of shoulder is negative pressure in glenoid cavity.
- Hanging cast is used for fracture shaft humerus
- Nerve involved in fracture shaft humerus is radial nerve
- Capitulum is the first epiphysis to appear around the elbow region
- Three point bony relationship is measured in 90 degrees flexion of elbow and it is maintained in supracondylar fracture humerus.
- The commonest type of supracondylar fracture is extension type and most common nerve involved is Anterior interosseous nerve>Median nerve.
- Gunstock deformity is cubitus varus seen in malunion of supracondylar fracture humerus.
- French osteotomy is done for cubitus varus

- Tardy ulnar nerve palsy is seen in cubitus valgus deformity.
- Lateral condyle humerus fracture complications are-Nonunion, Tardy ulnar nerve palsy and cubitus valgus deformity.
- Medial epicondyle fracture humerus ulnar nerve is involved.
- In Hansen's disease ulnar nerve is involved at elbow.
- Myositis ossificans is heterotopic bone formation and in acute stages it is treated by immobilization.
- Volkmann's ischemia first sign is Pain.
- In Volkmann's ischemic contracture commonest muscle involved is FDP (Flexor Digitorum Profundus) and commonest nerve involved are Anterior interossei >median nerve.
- Terrible triad of Elbow is Elbow dislocation with radial head and coronoid fracture.
- Elbow dislocation complications are vascular injury, Median nerve injury and VIC.
- While using crutches elbow should be flexed to 30 degrees.
- Monteggia fracture is fracture of upper ulna with dislocated radial head
- Mason's classification is for radial head fracture.
- Colle's fracture there is posterior displacement, lateral displacement, impaction and supination.
- Colle's fracture undergoes malunion into dinner fork deformity (it never undergoes nonunion or delayed union)
- Extensor pollicis longus tendon may be involved in Colle's fracture.
- Colle's fracture is treated by hand shaking cast
- Sudeck's dystrophy is most commonly seen in Colle's fracture. (Sudeck's dystrophy clinical features include-red hot shiny skin, patchy osteopenia after Colle's fracture)
- Allen's test is for radial artery
- Scaphoid fracture has tenderness in anatomical snuff box, blood supply comes in scaphoid from distal pole.
- Scaphoid fracture is treated by glass holding cast.
- Terry Thomas sign is seen in Carpal instability.
- Thoracic spine injury has maximum chances of paraplegia
- Railway spine is sequelae of railway accidents
- Hangman's fracture is fracture of C2 vertebrae

- Membranous part of urethra is damaged in fracture Pelvis
- Waddling gait is seen in bilateral Developmental dysplasia of hip.
- Trendelenberg test tests superior gluteal nerve and hip abductors (gluteus medius and minimus)
- Bryant's triangle measures supratrochanteric shortening and can find out damage to proximal femoral area and hip.
- Hemireplacement arthroplasty (Austin Moore replacement) is done for fracture neck femur >65 years of age.
- McMurray's osteotomy is done for fracture neck femur and is based on biomechanical principles.
- Intertrochanteric fracture neck femur there is external rotation of lower limb >45 degrees
- Pauwels' classification is for fracture neck of femur.
- Fracture neck of femur there is external rotation of <45 degrees.
- Posterior dislocation of hip there is Flexion, adduction and internal rotation.
- Posterior dislocation of Hip Femoral Artery pulsations are not felt (Vascular sign of Narath is positive)
- Femoral head with neck fracture is Pipkins type 3.
- Straddle fracture involves superior and inferior pubic rami.
- Supracondylar fracture femur can cause damage to popliteal artery
- Most dangerous complication of a long bone fracture is fat embolism
- Knee effusion is tested by patellar tap /fluctuation and filling of lateral fossae of knee.
- Patella commonly dislocates laterally
- 'Q' angle is increased in patella subluxation
- Bumper fracture involves lateral condyle of tibia
- Lisfrancs dislocation involves tarsometatarsal area
- Ideal treatment for fracture patella is tension band wiring
- March fracture is fracture of 2nd metatarsal neck
- Stress fracture most commonly involves metatarsals
- Runners fracture is fracture of lower end of fibula
- Bumper fracture involves lateral condyle of tibia
- Vessel injury in open fracture is Gustilo Anderson Grade 3C.

- Chauffeur's fracture involves radial styloid
- Barton's fracture involves fracture distal end radius with wrist subluxation
- Time taken for fractures to unite are transverse> oblique> spiral
- Open reduction in children is required for lateral condyle humerus fracture
- Ideal site for bone grafting is iliac crest

Maximum Weight for Skeletal Traction is 20 kg

K-wire is used for circlage and forearm bone fixation

Tension band wiring is done for fracture patella and olecranon

Non dynamic splint is cock up splint

Gallows traction is used for fracture shaft femur <2 years of age

Fracture shaft femur <5 years of age spica is treatment of choice.

Adult patient fracture shaft femur is treated by intramedullary nailing.

Intertrochanteric fracture is treated by Dynamic Hip Screw

Mallet finger is avulsion of base of distal phalanx

Medial collateral ligament injury is diagnosed by valgus stress test

McMurray's test is done for medial meniscus

Locking of knee is seen in bucket handle tear of meniscus

Lachman and anterior drawer test is for Anterior cruciate ligament.

Anterior cruciate ligament prevents anterior dislocation of tibia.

NEUROMUSCULAR DISORDERS

- Compound palmar ganglion has hourglass swelling that goes beneath flexor retinaculum
- Spondylolysis there is break in pars interarticularis
- Spondylolisthesis there is shift of one vertebra over the other and most common level is l5-S1
- Most common disc prolapse is L4-L5
- Tennis elbow there is lateral epicondylitis.
- Nursemaids elbow (Pulled elbow) there is Radial head subluxation
- De Quervain's tenosynovitis involves Abductor pollicis longus and extensor pollicis brevis (1st extensor compartment of wrist) and Finkelstein test is done for it.

- Muscles in 2nd compartment of wrist are ECRL/ECRB.
- Dupuytrens contracture involves ring finger > little finger, seen in cirrhosis, Table top test is positive and clostridial collagenase is used for treatment.
- Housemaids knee is pre patellar bursitis.
- Clergyman's knee is infra patellar bursitis
- Spring ligament is involved in pes planus
- Jones operation is for claw hallux.
- Keller's surgery is for hallux Valgus.

NERVE INJURIES

- Neurapraxia is physiological block in nerve conduction
- Tinel's sign is done for nerve regeneration and normal rate of nerve recovery is 1mm/day or 1 inch/month. Tinel's sign is positive and progressive in axonotmesis
- Motor march is seen in axonotmesis
- Median nerve supplies nail bed of middle finger
- Pointing index, Pen test and Benediction test are for Median nerve palsy
- Froment's sign is a feature of ulnar nerve palsy
- Ulnar nerve supplies Flexor digitorum profundus (medial half) and adductor pollicis
- Claw hand is called as main in griffe
- Knuckle bender splint is used for claw hand (ulnar nerve palsy>median nerve palsy)
- Total claw hand is seen in ulnar and median nerve palsy and partial claw hand in ulnar nerve palsy.
- Cock up splint is used for radial nerve palsy
- Sciatic nerve injury most common cause is traumatic> iatrogenic
- Fibular neck fracture causes palsy of Common Peroneal Nerve.
- Foot drop is seen in Sciatic nerve injury, injury to ankle dorsiflexors and Common peroneal nerve palsy.
- Sural nerve is most commonly used for nerve graft
- Carpal tunnel syndrome median nerve is involved
- Cubital tunnel syndrome ulnar nerve is involved

- Tarsal tunnel syndrome posterior tibial nerve is involved
- Guyon's canal ulnar nerve is involved
- Hand knee gait is seen in polio
- Foot drop -posterior tibial tendon is transferred to dorsum of foot.
- Erb's palsy there is upper trunk -C5-C6 nerve root involvement
- Erb's palsy there is policeman or waiters tip deformity- there is loss of abduction and external rotation of shoulder, flexion of elbow and supination of forearm.
- Splint used for brachial plexus injury is Aeroplane splint.
- Winging of scapula is seen in injury to long thoracic nerve.

JOINT DISORDERS

- HLA B 27 is associated with Ankylosing spondylitis
- Ankylosing spondylitis there is sacroiliac involvement and there is a Bamboo spine.
- Knee is the most common joint involved in osteoarthritis of knee and medial compartment is involved.
- Quadriceps femoris is main extensor of knee joint
- Distal Inter Phalangeal involvement causes Heberden nodes in Osteoarthritis
- Osteoarthritis usually does not involve coracoclavicular joint.
- Metacarpophalangeal involvement is seen in Rheumatoid arthritis and there is sparing of DIP.
- Swan neck deformity is seen in Rheumatoid arthritis it involves flexion at DIP and hyperextension at PIP.
- Boutonniere deformity is also seen in Rheumatoid arthritis and it involves hyperextension at DIP and flexion at PIP.
- C1-C2 involvement is seen in Rheumatoid arthritis
- Gout uric acid crystals are deposited
- DOC acute attach NSAIDS.
- Pseudogout there is calcium pyrophosphate crystal deposition
- Charcots joints most commonly occurs in Diabetes mellitus and it usually involves foot area
- Intra-articular calcification is seen in Charcots joints
- Osteoarthritis of hip is treated by Total Hip Replacement

- OA hip in elderly cemented Total Hip Replacement is done.
- Osteoarthritis of knee limiting activities of daily living affected is treated by Total Knee Replacement
- Thalassemia involves knee joint.

METABOLIC BONE DISORDERS

- Osteomalacia has proximal myopathy, loosers zones and triradiate pelvis.
- Alkaline phosphatase is high in rickets and osteomalacia. The value of ALP is normal in osteoporosis and Multiple myeloma.
- Frankel's line and Wimbergers ring sign are seen in scurvy
- Stoss therapy is for rickets
- Cupping of bone ends, beading of costochondral junction and genu varum is seen in rickets
- Arachnodactyly is seen in Marfan's syndrome
- Short 4th and 5th metacarpal is seen in pseudohypoparathyroidism
- Codfish vertebra are seen in osteoporosis
- Hyperparathyroidism there is subperiosteal resorption in phalanges.
- Marble bone appearance is seen in osteopetrosis (osteoclast defect)
- Bone within bone appearance is seen in osteopetrosis
- Relentless pain in Paget's disease is due to Malignant degeneration, pathological fracture and osteoarthritis.
- Clutton's joints are seen in late congenital syphilis
- Postmenopausal osteoporosis bisphosphonates are used.

PEDIATRIC ORTHOPEDICS

- Manus valgus is due to absent radius.
- Perthes disease is osteochondritis of femoral epiphysis (Avascular necrosis of femoral head)
- Kienbock's disease is avascular necrosis (osteochondritis) of lunate
- Salter-Harris classification is for epiphyseal injuries in children
- Thurston Holland sign is for type 2 Salter-Harris injury.

- Rocker bottom foot is seen in congenital vertical talus and incorrect correction of CTEV.
- Ortolani and Barlow test is for DDH
- DDH brace -Von Rosen splint and Pawlik harness.
- Splint for Perthes disease is Scottish Rite.
- Idiopathic scoliosis is for lateral curvature of spine with rotational component.
- Splint used for scoliosis is Milwaukee brace and Boston brace
- Triple arthrodesis involves talonavicular, talocalcaneal and calcaneocuboid fusion.
- Duchenne muscular dystrophy there is involvement of calf muscle causing pseudohypertrophy and there is Gowers sign.
- Dynamisation of nail is done for delayed union of bones
- Forearm fracture in 5 year old child is treated by reduction and cast.
- Avascular necrosis is seen in femoral head, scaphoid, talus and lunate. It is associated with steroid intake, alcohol intake or patient on dialysis. Investigation of choice is MRI.
- Cluttons joint is seen in late congonital syphilis.
- Trethovan sign is used in slipped capital femoral epiphysis.
- Fairbank's triangle is seen in coxa vora.

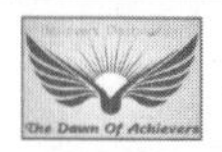

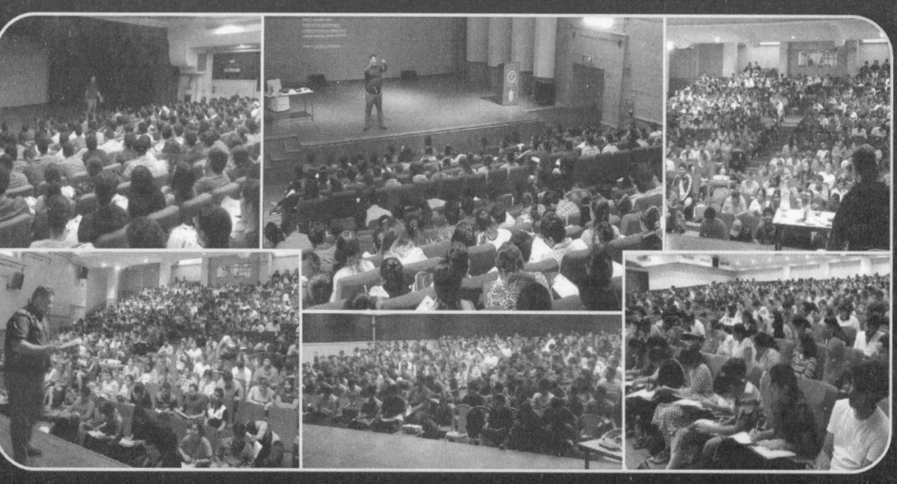

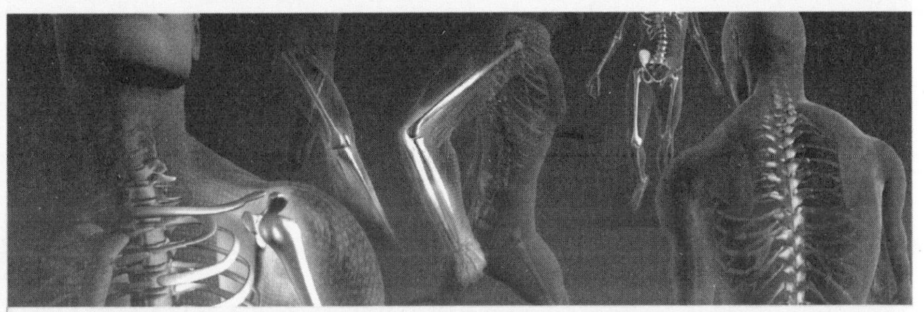

ORTHOPEDICS SIMPLIFIED

for Undergraduate

Apurv Mehra

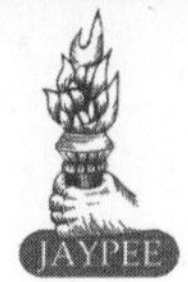